Natural Childbirth
and
the Family

Natural Childbirth and the Family

Revised Edition

Helen Wessel

Harper & Row, Publishers

New York, Evanston, San Francisco, London

This book was originally published under the title *Natural Childbirth and the Christian Family*.

Excerpt on page 282 from *Modern Motherhood: Revised Edition* by H. M. I. Liley, M.D., with Beth Day. Copyright © 1969 by Beth Day.

Excerpt on page 280 from *Why Natural Childbirth?* by Deborah Tanzer, Ph.D., and Jean L. Block. Published by Doubleday & Company, Inc.

NATURAL CHILDBIRTH AND THE FAMILY, Revised Edition. Copyright © 1963, 1973 by Helen S. Wessel. All rights reserved. Printed in the United States of America. No part of this book may be used or reproduced in any manner whatsoever without written permission except in the case of brief quotations embodied in critical articles and reviews. For information address Harper & Row, Publishers, Inc., 10 East 53rd Street, New York, N.Y. 10022. Published simultaneously in Canada by Fitzhenry & Whiteside Limited, Toronto.

Design by Janice Stern

Library of Congress Cataloging in Publication Data
Wessel, Helen (Strain) 1924-
    Natural childbirth and the family.
    First ed. published in 1963 under title: Natural childbirth and the Christian family.
    Bibliography: p.
    1. Childbirth—Psychology.   I. Title.
[DNLM: 1. Natural childbirth.   WQ150 W511n 1974]
RG661.W45   1974   618.4'5   73-4136
ISBN 0-06-014542-0

This book is lovingly dedicated to my sons
and daughters and their sons and daughters.

Contents

Acknowledgments

Many people have contributed in many ways to this book. It is not possible to thank them all by name, but I would like to express my appreciation to the following persons:

To my husband, *Walter W. Wessel,* Ph.D., for his constant praise, encouragement, and helpful criticisms. He has never discouraged my searching for answers in the areas in which, as a Biblical and linguistic scholar, he is the expert and I am the novice. He has patiently corrected my mistakes, and placed all his resources for Biblical research freely at my disposal.

To my father, *John Albert Strain,* for the use of his poems "The Sculptor" and "The Rock," and for designing the portable back rest which may be used on delivery tables or for home births. Most of all, I am grateful to him for having taught me, by the example of his life, the lesson of implicit faith in a loving God.

To the late *Dr. Grantly Dick-Read,* whom I was never privileged to meet but whose teachings confirmed my intuitive belief from childhood that the goodness of God is not limited in its expression in any area of our lives—not even in the experience of giving birth.

To *Minnie Sue Buckingham,* Ph.D., for her stimulating teaching of literature and creative writing, and for her personal friendship and encouragement through the years.

To *Harold E. Grove*, my editor at Harper & Row, for his helpful co-operation and prompt attention to every question, and for demonstrating the warm friendliness that keeps this publishing house from being a big, impersonal business.

To *Carol Nelson*, for her beautiful line drawings which illustrate the book.

To *Sister Mary Meyer*, obstetric supervisor at St. Joseph's Hospital, St. Paul, Minnesota, for her dedication to family-centered maternity care in the hospital setting, and for the inspiration of her continuing efforts for community-wide childbirth education.

To *Ilene Rice*, breast-feeding consultant at St. Joseph's Hospital, and mother of three children, for contributing the helpful material included in the chapter "Breast-Feeding."

To *Donald Singerman*, librarian of the Mount Zion Temple library, St. Paul, for his patient, friendly assistance in locating necessary Jewish source material.

Foreword

This is an unusual book and one that should be read by prospective mothers and their doctors.

Here one finds an unusual blending of Christian faith and principles of medical truth in a woefully neglected or flouted area. The arguments and experience of the author will stand up from a scriptural standpoint and in the clear light of professional practice.

The author knows how to write, has deep Christian convictions, and at the same time presents her thesis in terms laymen and doctors can understand and follow to great profit.

It is our hope that this book will have the circulation it deserves —with prospective parents, with doctors in the specialized field of obstetrics, and with pastors for whom it also has a message. It will prove a rewarding concept of the problems they all face.

L. NELSON BELL, M.D., F.A.C.S.

Preface

Giving birth is one of the most beautiful spiritual and physical experiences woven into the tapestry of a woman's life. This has been proven in the lives of many thousands of women like myself, who have had the privilege of giving birth to babies naturally. By following the teachings of the late Dr. Grantly Dick-Read, the great pioneer of the natural-childbirth philosophy, we have found it true that childbirth is a normal physiological function of the human body and is not meant to be painful.

Dr. Dick-Read's kind heart was touched in his early days of medical practice when he observed the pain of women in labor—women who were suffering in spite of all the medication and relief that science had to offer. He dedicated his life to research for ways to prevent this pain by natural means, rather than by attempting to blot it out with ineffective, dangerous drugs. He searched for normal, common-sense ways it could be prevented, because he had faith that God did not intend women to suffer in childbirth. He followed this leading of his heart to success. Our society owes grateful tribute to the memory of his dedicated life.

Giving birth to a child is a "natural" event, but one must learn how to work in harmony with the processes of "nature," just as it is necessary to learn the basic principles of good health. Adequate prenatal education for both husband and wife is necessary. Relaxation and breathing must be properly learned during pregnancy. Support should be given the mother in labor and delivery by her husband, as well as by medical attendants, and the mother should learn in advance how she can "give birth" actively, and happily, rather than being passively "delivered."

Because of the importance of maintaining a warm and understanding relationship between husband and wife during labor and birth, as well as during courtship, marriage, pregnancy, and parenthood, this book emphasizes "family-centered" maternity care. After all, God did not create human life to exist in a vacuum, but invented the first "family" concept.

The material presented is given in two parts. First the "story" of John and Mary, who demonstrate by example wholesome attitudes toward sex, marriage, and the birth of a child. The story form is used to make the material more easily understood. It should be noted, however, that the labor and birth experiences of the young wife and her friend are not "idealistic fiction," but are based on the actual experiences of women bearing their first child, women I have known personally.

The second part of this book consists of more detailed discussion than is possible in the story, and will be helpful not only to young couples, but also to the doctors, nurses, pastors, educators, and others who have the responsibility of counseling them.

Many have asked how I became interested in natural childbirth and if all our children were born in this way. My own deep concern over current childbirth practices occurred as the result of my suffering at the birth of our third child. I had not been happy about the births of our first two children, but did nothing about it.

When our first child was born, I was completely anesthetized for the birth, without any warning that this would take place. I awakened from the anesthetic angry and disappointed that I had been denied the right to be present at the birth of my own child, an experience I had looked forward to with keen anticipation. I expected to breast-feed my baby, but she was never brought to me. Finally, I asked a nurse, "Why don't they bring me my baby to breast-feed?"

She gave me a startled look, and then said, "You can't breast-feed your baby," and left. When the doctor came in, I asked the same question and received a similar answer, with no explanation. This surprising disappointment was so upsetting that I cried all night.

Labor for our second daughter began with gentle, regular contractions. The doctor examined me on my arrival at the hospital, and I was suddenly startled by a rush of water. "I just ruptured the membranes," he explained, "to speed things up." I was deeply annoyed, but it was too late to object. Heavy medication kept me asleep during labor, but I awakened to find myself bearing down hard, was taken to the delivery room and given a spinal anesthetic.

What a joy to be awake to see my daughter's little body lifted up before my own eyes! But my lower body was as void of sensation as if it were dead. The paralysis lasted for long hours, until I began to wonder if I could ever move my legs again. "Does it sometimes happen," I asked the nurse, "that one can become permanently paralyzed by a spinal anesthetic?"

"Hush," she whispered. "We don't talk about such things here!"

For days following the birth my head ached whenever I raised it from the pillow. I was informed that this was a common after-effect of spinal anesthesia.

No women in this hospital were allowed to breast-feed their babies, for an epidemic had occurred earlier in the year in a nearby hospital in which twenty-five babies died in a week. Thus all babies were kept in the nurseries continually until discharge. The first time I held this little daughter was the day we left the hospital.

Three years later I was back in the hospital—for extensive cervical repair of damage caused by the birth—and was discharged three days later. The cervical damage may have been partly due to the premature rupture of the membranes and to the fact that I was bearing down under sedation, no doubt before the cervix was dilated. Whatever the cause, it was left unrepaired at the time of the birth. The physician who repaired it said I would never have been able to carry a fetus longer than three months without the repair.

The third pregnancy was complicated by threatened premature labor from the fifth month on, so that every few days I had to go to bed under strong medication to quiet the restless uterus. My physician was highly qualified and kind, insisting that I call him any time of the day or night when contractions began and that I not take any medication to stop them without his express permission. Under his conscientious care I kept the baby until full term, though physically and emotionally exhausted from the long months of anxiety. It was a great relief when labor began, and I walked confidently into the most excruciatingly painful and shocking experience of my life.

The labor was brief, with powerful, almost continuous contractions that seemed to accomplish nothing. Suddenly, while still alone in the room, the cervical scar tissue violently ruptured. Nurses came running, dashed me down the hall on a gurney and onto the delivery table. A saddle block was given, my hands and legs strapped down, and a blindfold and oxygen mask clamped over my face. But the saddle block had no time to take effect, and as the birth began I experienced the most blinding pain I have ever known. My screams were totally ignored, and as the intensity of pain increased I lost consciousness. When I came to shortly after, those around me were talking nonchalantly as if nothing had happened!

The mask was removed, I was shown the baby, the doctor prepared to repair the episiotomy, and then said softly under his breath, "My gosh! We're going to be here all night!" But after forty-five minutes of patient stitching he finished the repair and I was taken to my room, still stunned and in a state of shock. My husband came beaming into the room, leaned over and said, "The doctor tells me you had a *very easy delivery*. I'm so glad!" I stared at him in astonishment, and then closed my eyes without answering until he went away. It was as if a curtain had fallen between me and every other human being, even the one I loved best.

For days I was too weak to lift my head, turn myself in bed without assistance, or even eat, for a fork was too heavy to hold. There was no question of breast feeding this baby, for I didn't even want to see her bruised and swollen face. One day, when the nurse brought her to the room for me to see, I said, "Please, not today," and turned away.

"You don't want your *baby*?" she asked indignantly.

"No," I whispered. She marched away, her footsteps echoing down the long hallway. Then, for the first time, I cried. Tears of shame and guilt rolled down my cheeks, into my ears, and splashed onto the pillow. I didn't even want my own baby! I felt too wicked even to pray.

A little Mexican grandmother came softly into the room, pushing a dustmop. Noticing my tears, she came near the bed and laid her hand tenderly on my leg. Tears of sympathy rolled down her own brown, wrinkled cheeks as she stood there several moments without a word. She may have known no English, but love has a language of its own, and I was comforted, drawn back into the world of human beings who understood. As my tears ceased, she slipped away as quietly as she had come. I never saw her again, but I have thanked God for her ever since.

Not until years later did I learn that the terrible pain had been caused by forceps the doctor was using to control the birth—my flesh crushed painfully between steel and bone, while he assumed the area was anesthetized and ignored my cries because he believed I was "asleep." No one had meant to be unkind.

The following weeks and months were frightening because my strength returned so slowly and I was losing weight continually. I was too ill to give the baby more than minimal care for a long time, and she spent a large part of every day propped up on her daddy's shoulder. If I passed a store window with a man inside wearing a white coat—even a barber—I would break into a sweat and begin trembling all over. Even God seemed changed—not the loving God I had always known but an angry God who had damned half the world to such suffering. It just couldn't be. God was not like that. Questions flooded my mind, demanding answers. If mine had been an "easy" birth, what indeed must a "hard" one be? If I was fortunate, as the doctor had said, to have had such excellent medical attention, what indeed must be the plight of the unaided woman?

Then, one day, stepping into the yard, I noticed for the first time that the trees were still green, the sky was still blue. How strange. It seemed that everything should be different, for God was not the loving Saviour I had known so intimately before. On returning indoors, I picked up a hymnal at random and flipped it open. "O

God, our help in ages past, Our hope for years to come,"—the words leaped out before my startled eyes:

> Before the hills in order stood
> Or earth received her frame,
> From everlasting Thou art God,
> From age to age the same.

God had not changed. Why then—blasphemous thought—had He deserted me and not helped me in my desperate need? One day I picked up my Bible, and God spoke to me unexpectedly in the words of Isaiah 54:8:

> For a small moment have I forsaken thee; but with great mercies will I gather thee. In a little wrath I hid my face from thee for a moment; but with everlasting kindness will I have mercy on thee, saith the Lord my Redeemer.

God had permitted this to happen, and had a purpose in it for me. It was not "meaningless" suffering. My responsibility now was to find His purpose, so that the experience could be used to honor Him and prevent such terrible suffering for others. Prayerfully I began searching the Scriptures day after day to find the answers. At first fearful of what I might find, I was delightfully surprised again and again. God is indeed the loving Saviour, the Creator who does all things well. The wonderful Biblical truths I discovered are all recorded in this book.

One day, while I was learning these things, God brought into my hands *Childbirth Without Fear* by Grantly Dick-Read. I wept all the way through the book. Here at last was a doctor who understood how a woman feels. Here was a man whose teaching was in harmony with what God was showing me in the Bible. Though still badly frightened, I was determined to have another baby as soon as possible, to discover for myself if these truths were really so. My sanity and my faith depended upon their validity.

My pregnancy had just begun when a letter came, saying that my young cousin Ruth had died at the birth of her first child. It seemed incredible. Ruth, so radiantly healthy and happy—who of all persons would have wanted a natural birth if she had known it was possible—was gone. Just before the birth she had been routinely put under anesthesia, although she had not made one sound of complaint during her entire labor, nor had she asked for an anesthetic. Under anesthesia she vomited, her jaws locked, her throat constricted, the fluid went into her lungs and shut off the air. She never regained consciousness or ever saw her baby, though the doctor tried valiantly for four hours to restore a normal heart-beat. The doctor said she had had "an easy delivery." Easy for whom? Ruth was dead.

It was at this time that I first wrote Dr. Dick-Read, for reassurance, and sent him a treatise I had written called "The Biblical Teaching Concerning Labor and Childbirth." I received a long, beautiful letter in reply. This was the beginning of a cherished correspondence. In one letter he said,

> . . . I am making a big effort to have the prayer book of the English Church changed. Their service for the Churching of Women, which is ostensibly to give thanks for the birth of the child, is one of the most heretical misinterpretations of truth I have ever read, and it offends me when women come to me and say, "Yes, I went to Church, but I didn't repeat the service because it wasn't true." I have heard that many times in my life. . . .

Our fourth daughter was born one beautiful Sunday in December, 1954, six weeks prematurely. I had noticed contractions during the morning at church and called the doctor about noon, after having gone right to bed and relaxing completely for a while to see if the contractions would go away. He asked, "Do the contractions hurt?" When I told him I could tell I was having a contraction only by placing my hand on my abdomen, because I was so relaxed, he said, "It's probably only false labor. Call me later if it doesn't stop."

Contractions were already only three and a half minutes apart, but I lay down again, becoming as limp as possible to *stop* labor if possible, and keep the baby until full term. But each time I touched my abdomen to see if I was having a contraction, it was hard beneath my fingers. Suddenly, at four o'clock, I realized that not only was I really in labor—the baby would soon be born! We got to the hospital, and I was quickly taken to the delivery room. My husband had been promised he could be with me, but since our doctor was not there, he was shut out by the nurse. The baby was born at 4:20 P.M., so gently that the water sac had not even broken, and had to be punctured by the attendant. More remarkable still was that the badly scarred, irregular cervix had received no further injury. My doctor, red-faced, came flying into the room a couple of moments after the baby had arrived.

I felt so marvelous, so elated, I could have picked up my baby and walked back home! But one look at my husband's long face a few minutes later, and I said to myself, "I will *never* have another baby in the hospital. This is one disappointment too many." We named our beautiful little daughter Dorothy, which means "the gift of God," for indeed she was. I wanted another baby as soon as possible.

Fourteen months later our first son was born at home—the most beautiful experience of my life. I planned the circumstances carefully in advance and made a back rest for myself. Only the doctor and my husband were present, while the other children were sent to the neighbors for a short time. There was no pain, or hurry, and the baby arrived in an atmosphere of dignity and peace. Afterward, I felt so refreshed and exuberant that I got up, took care of the baby myself, combed my hair and put the room back in order. And then, because it seemed to be the thing to do, I lay down again, although I felt absolutely marvelous. I feasted my eyes on this precious baby all day long.

For the birth of our sixth child, another son, five years later, I returned to the hospital for the birth, on one condition—that my husband be with me the entire time. The attendants were most co-operative and it was a beautiful birth, marred only by the discomfort of not having a back rest on the delivery table and breast engorgement from not being able to breast-feed on demand. A few weeks later a breast infection and kidney infection developed from the hospital stay, and though my recovery was uneventful, the baby refused to breast-feed on the side that had been affected. I had successfully breast-fed the first two "natural babies," so I continued feeding this one for several months on the breast he would accept, and he thrived.

To every John and Mary who reads this book, looking forward to sharing one of the most precious of life's experiences—the birth of a little son or daughter—I would say:

Faith is the secret of success: faith in the rightness and beauty of conception and birth; faith in a loving God who made our bodies as they are. Rest on this faith when labor begins, relax all tensions and cares and wait patiently for love's reward.

HELEN WESSEL

Part I

Chapter 1

The Way of a Man with a Maid

Whoso findeth a wife findeth a good thing, and
obtaineth favour of the Lord. Prov. 18:22.

Twilight slowly wrapped the world with silent fingers as the long shadows of the cedars and pines crept stealthily up the hillside, thrown into silhouettes by the setting sun. John and Mary paused a moment in their walk to watch its final burst of glory before it slipped out of sight behind the blue Pacific. The only sound to be heard was the distant, rhythmic rumble of the surf, and Mary gave a little start when John broke the silence suddenly.

"We'd better be getting back. It'll be dark soon, and there are no paths near us here."

"Just a minute, honey. It's so beautiful now. See that little cloud just above the horizon? It reminds me of the poem I wrote in high school, 'The Maiden.' "

" 'The Maiden'? Hey, that sounds interesting. I like maidens, especially this one! Remember what Solomon said? 'There be three things which are too wonderful for me, yea, four which I know not: The way of . . .' "

"John! Be serious a moment! I'm not talking about *that* kind of maiden. I'm talking about, well—nature—you know, that sort of thing."

"That's right, I married a poet, didn't I? Okay, let's hear this nature thing, or whatever it is."

3

"John!"

"I'm only teasing, honey. C'mon, let's hear it."

John watched his darling as she recited her little creation, more fascinated by the soft curves of her cheek and chin in the growing dusk than in what she was reciting to him—

> In the solemn stillness of an early dawn is heard
>   The crystal-throated reveille of a waking bird.
> Donning golden slippers arises then the Day
>   And flings across the morning sky her crimson negligee.
>
> Enchanting now, she saunters forth to spread abroad her
>   charm
>   And shakes perfume from every flower to smooth upon
>   her arm.
> She paints the children's bodies brown, their faces rosy fair,
>   And with soft fluting of the wind breathes kisses through
>   their hair.
>
> Shrill piccolo of the cricket warns that night at last has
>   come!
>   She gathers up her flowing skirts and hastens quickly
>   home.
> But looking up into the sky, a wary child might find—
>   She left her veil of mauve chiffon trailing far behind.

"Mary, that's beautiful! You know what? You can write all the poetry you like—just so you learn to sew on a button, fry an egg, and a few irrelevant, mundane things."

Mary gave her head a little toss as she turned away, pretending to be cross. "That just shows what *you* are. You may think I'm an unrealistic, dreaming poet, but I think you're a preacher!"

Laughingly they turned and started arm in arm down the hillside toward their little cottage, delighted not so much with their own joking as with the fun of knowing that they were going to be together for ever and ever.

The day of the wedding had been sunny and warm. There had been a good many misgivings in Mrs. Johnson's mind about the feasibility of an outdoor wedding, knowing the fickleness of the weather, even in early June. She had been anxious to please her daughter, but all the same she had planned how she would manage indoors in case of rain. The tears came to her eyes as she pictured what a lovely bride her Mary had been, moving gracefully over the lawn on her father's arm to the little bower that had been arranged for the altar.

"It seems so right, Mother," Mary had told her earlier, "that we should be married out of doors. God's world is so beautiful. I don't see how we could ever decorate a church to look half so nice. Remember the time I wrote that poem about the world being like a cathedral?"

Mrs. Johnson remembered all right. She had saved every scrap of her daughter's poetic scribblings—had them tucked away in a special box. She lifted her hands out of the dishwater a moment and smiled to herself as she thought of one of Mary's birthday poems for her, carefully decorated with a drawing of a very lop-sided blue cake—

> I love you Mother More and more
> Even though Your thirty four.

How old was Mary then. Eight? Nine? Well, it didn't matter, only it seemed such a short time ago.

And it seemed such a short while since the starlit night when they had been driving home from a day at the seashore. Jo Lynn was asleep in the back seat, and Mary was snuggled in the front seat with them. Suddenly she had whispered, "Look, Mama 'n' Daddy—the sky has on its polka-dot pajamas!"

Jo Lynn had been a pretty bridesmaid too. I'm fortunate to have such beautiful daughters, Mrs. Johnson thought. Unless I'm prejudiced. But they really *are* pretty, even though Jo Lynn is so different, athletic and jolly, like her Dad. It's a good thing she saw where the ring rolled when Paulie dropped it! We never would have found it in the grass otherwise.

Absently Mrs. Johnson wiped her hands on the dish towel before sitting down a moment, engrossed now in the scene of the wedding. It was just like Mary, she thought, to turn a wee bit farther toward us when she recited her verse to John, so Grandma could hear her clearly too—

> John, 'whither thou goest, I will go; and where thou lodgest, I will lodge: thy people shall be my people, and thy God my God: the Lord do so to me, and more also, if ought but death part thee and me.'

There had been no danger of Grandma's not hearing John's reply, spoken with such profound sincerity! "Mary, I promise to love you and cherish you, even as Christ also loved the church, and gave himself for it!"

Mrs. Johnson's thoughts turned to the short wedding sermon on the founding of a godly home that Pastor Dirkson had given the young couple during the ceremony. She gratefully reviewed all that he had said and prayed in her heart that his words might become reality in John and Mary's lives.

"It was not the Creator's plan," the pastor had said, "for the people of the world to live alone, even though He created each one of us as a distinct individual. The Bible tells us that He brings joy to lonely hearts by setting 'the solitary in families.' When He created Adam, He said, 'It is not good that the man should be alone. . . .'

"God did not give Adam a family at once—just one person to meet his need. It is God who has put within our hearts this need to share with someone special our deepest thoughts and feelings and emotions. This 'someone special' is a person of the opposite sex, for 'male and female created he them'; the male all strength and masculinity, the female all feminine gentleness and beauty, each the complement of the other. Thus it was that Adam felt his loneliness, and Eve was given to him by the Creator to be his wife.

"Notice God's order in the establishing of the home: man was created first, then the woman. Now some have seemed to think that because of this order man is more important than woman and that she is an inferior creation. But if one is arguing of the importance of the *order* of creation, it is well to remember that God created the angels, and *every living creature as well* before He created man! Since we are clearly told in Corinthians that man is higher than the angels, if we are to use order as a sign of intrinsic worth, it will be necessary to conclude that in creating a lovely wife for Adam, God had saved the best for the last!

"The order of creation does not indicate the superiority or inferiority of man or woman but, rather, God's pattern for the harmonious functioning of a godly home. There is to be no competition between husband and wife but only a sense of completion and fulfillment. The husband is the head of the home, the protector and provider; the wife his helper and the keeper of the household. Both share in the responsibility of rearing children, as it says in Proverbs: 'My son, hear the instruction of thy father, and forsake not the law of thy mother.'

"Much unhappiness has arisen over a misunderstanding of God's plan. He did not intend that a man should 'lord it over' his wife or that she should be strictly limited to responsibilities within the home. Because of their intrinsic worth as individuals, each was to be free to develop his or her potential abilities to full capacity, secure and confident in their marriage relationship. It is sometimes overlooked that the description of the perfect wife in Proverbs 31 shows her to be a woman of many talents. Here she is not only industrious in the home, feeding and clothing her family, but we find her also in the market place selling her merchandise, in the countryside purchasing land, and among the poor 'reaching forth' her hands to the needy. She was free to use the talents God had given her. Because she really loved her husband, in renunciation of herself continually putting his needs and those of her children before her own, his heart safely trusted in her: 'Her children arise up, and call her blessed; her husband also, and he praiseth her.'

"Women have an instinctive, God-given desire to please their husbands and to look up to them. This is brought out at the beginning of our Bible, where it says of Eve in Genesis 3:16, 'her *desire* shall be to her husband.' The Hebrew word for 'desire' can also be translated as 'longing.' In a Greek translation of the Old Testament (the Septuagint) this phrase reads: *kai pros ton andra sou hē apostrophē sou* (your *turning* will be to your husband).

"How true to life it is that in the times of her deepest need a wife longs to turn to her husband, her guard and protector, for his love and sympathy. In the Song of Solomon there is a picture of this relationship between man and wife. 'I sat down under his shadow with great delight,' says the young br' !e, 'and his banner over me was love.'

"So do not be afraid, Mary, to submit to Jo.   s loving authority in the home, knowing that you are still free to develop fully as an individual. May your attitude toward him be as   you were to say, 'I am his willing helper. He has captured my devotion!'

"But what if you disagree with John on som. important matter, even after an honest discussion? The God-given principle is that you are to submit to his decision, even though you feel it is wrong. If instead you resist, either by silent resentment or by open anger and rebellion, your attitude will be destructive both to you as a person and to the marriage. Remember that you always have resource to a higher authority than John, so t .e your complaints freely to the Father in heaven, and let Him work out the problem.

"And, John, although in God's plan the husband is the head of the wife, remember that Paul goes on to say that this is to be 'even as Christ is the head of the church.' The 'headship' of Christ is not one of tyranny, or of domineering, but a rule of tenderness and concern. His example is that of a renunciation of Himself—a sacrificial and a giving love, *even to the point of death* for the sake of His bride, the Church. Surely no higher standard than this could be given for a husband's behavior toward his wife.

"Nor is this all. God has included in His plan for married love a sharing with Himself in the making of little children. Thus it is that when a child is born into the atmosphere of harmony and self-giving love of a godly home, we can see the beauty of the unfolding pattern of God's design: father, mother, child."

Bear and Forbear

Live together in harmony, live together in love, as though you had only one mind and one spirit between you. Never act from motives of rivalry or personal vanity, but in humility think more of each other than you do of yourselves. Phil. 2:2—3 (Phillips translation).

Mary quickly gathered up the breakfast dishes and carried them to the sink. She and John hoped to leave home while it was still early, since it might get quite hot on the road before they reached Uncle George's and Aunt Emma's.

"I'll be back in a few minutes, Mary," John called over his shoulder as he strode out to the car, letting the screen door bang behind him.

Now where is he going, Mary wondered, annoyed. She hurried to call after him, but John was already driving away. I suppose he wants to get something done to the car for the trip, or maybe get gasoline, she thought. At least he could have told me where he was going and not just go whamming out the door like that! We could just as well have stopped along the way somewhere.

Mary didn't fret long, however, since there was much to be done. She finished putting away the dishes, packed the bags, and cast a hurried glance through the rooms for anything she might have missed. John was still not back, so she stepped out the door onto the soft carpet of grass, inhaling deeply the delightfully refreshing fragrance of the evergreens, the trees she most loved. She stood quietly a few moments watching their stately branches feather-dusting the sky under the touch of a gentle breeze, enjoying a bird's song from somewhere in the branches. Her sensitive ear caught the rustling bustle of a little stream nearby. What a lovely place this was! She wished she had a piece of paper so she could jot down some of the phrases forming in her mind for a new poem.

The toothbrushes! she thought suddenly, and rushed back into the house. Sure enough, she had forgotten them. They still lay in patient repose on the window ledge of the little bathroom, for want of a better place. She had thought of them just in time, for the car was already turning into the lane.

"Ready?" John asked.

"Yes. Everything's all packed. Where have you been? You might at least have told me where you were going!" Mary didn't mean to sound cross, but she certainly did.

"Why, honey! I just went to get some gasoline while you got things gathered up. I thought it would save us some time. I'm sorry if I worried you."

"It's all right," Mary shrugged. "If you'll put the suitcases in the car, we can be on our way."

John obliged, and they were soon out on the highway. "You look so fresh and pretty this morning," John volunteered, hoping to make amends for offending his little bride. Mary had tucked a yellow ribbon in her hair, and did look charming.

"Thank you, John." Mary smoothed down the hem of her skirt and moved a bit closer to him.

"You sure you got everything, sweetheart?"

"Oh yes, I'm quite sure. I went all through the rooms again to be sure we didn't forget anything."

"You got my razor, I hope." John glanced at her anxiously.

"Your—razor? I don't quite remember—but I *did* go back through all the rooms—"

"You don't remember! We'd better stop and be sure." John

pulled over to the side of the road. Several minutes of shuffling through the carefully packed bags were of no avail.

"But, honey, I'm *sure*—"

"You may be sure, Mary, but it's not here. We'll have to go back. I can't get along without my razor—what do you expect me to do? Scrape my chin with a paring knife?"

Mary's eyes filled with tears, and she sat quietly the twenty miles back to the house. If only she had checked through it more carefully, rather than wasting so much time outdoors!

"I'm sorry, John. I really am."

"It's all right, honey. I didn't mean to be cross." John pulled her over near him, ignoring the hazards of one-arm driving. "We'll just enjoy the extra traveling time together. I guess I can't expect my little wife to remember all my stuff until I've been around a while longer.—And I mean to be around a *long, long time.*"

They drove in silence for a few minutes, when a thought suddenly occurred to John. He glanced over at Mary with a sly grin and asked impishly, "By the way, write any poems this morning?"

"No!" Mary said, half truthfully. She turned away to look out the car window so he could not see the guilty color rising in her cheeks.

"This was sure a good idea, Mary." John reached into the grocery bag for the Cokes. "Would you hand me the bottle opener for a moment?"

Mary was spreading the plastic picnic cloth on the grass just off the highway. "It's a good thing you spotted that store back there, John. I was beginning to think we weren't going to find anything open. I like this so much better than eating indoors—we can be by ourselves, and can walk around a bit. What are you smiling about?" she wondered, as she happened to notice his amused expression.

"H'm? Oh, I was thinking of the lady who played the organ in the little chapel we visited last month."

"She was a riot, all right," Mary agreed. "She was so short and fat I don't see how she could manage the pedals at all. It didn't seem to matter to her how many notes she missed, just so she impressed everyone by playing as loud and as fast as she could. It almost spoiled the service for me." Mary handed John a sandwich on a napkin, and they both sat down.

"Thanks, honey." John munched on his sandwich a while as he studied the landscape around them. "I don't know what made me think of the organist," he said between mouthfuls, "unless it's the way this spot reminds me of the chapel. Notice the hill sloping down toward the water fountain"—he gestured, with a sweep of his arm—"the way the hill sloped down toward the pulpit in the chapel. And the logs set around here for benches are the same kind, only here they're put every which way, not in neat rows."

"I loved the service," Mary reminisced with him, "except for the organist. I liked what the minister said about the God of Creation also being a God of love."

"I appreciated the sermon too, Mary. To think that God is interested in every little detail of our lives! I don't think I ever heard anyone preach on the 145th Psalm before, but the contrast is there all right!—the mighty God where it says 'Great is the Lord, . . . and his greatness is unsearchable'; and then the gentle and loving God where it says 'The Lord is good to all: and his tender mercies are over all his works.' "

"I liked what he said about God's perfect love casting out fear of a terrible God," Mary added.

"So did I—especially the way he compared this to the Israelites at Sinai who thought that the God of Creation was so powerful and so dreadful that they were afraid to come near Him, with the fact that Jesus came to show us God is Love, and to take away all our fear."

Mary was gathering things up as he spoke. "Hadn't we better be on our way, John? It's getting late."

Uncle George and Aunt Emma kept going to the door and looking down the road in anticipation of their young guests. But the tranquil silence of the late summer afternoon was interrupted only by the lowing of a cow in the pasture. And if it had not been for the occasional ambling of a heifer in search of a more choice morsel of grass, the scene just beyond their doorway would have been as motionless as a water-color in a frame.

"They're coming, George!" Aunt Emma called suddenly, as the car came into view down the road. Uncle George eased himself out of his rocking chair and came to wait beside her.

"Hello, Uncle George 'n' Aunt Em," John called gaily as he stepped out of the car. "Look what I've brought to show off to you!" He helped Mary from the car and drew her toward them. "This is my wife, Mary. Mary, this is Uncle George and Aunt Em."

"We're *so* glad to have you, Mary," Aunt Emma said warmly, putting out her hand to draw Mary's arm through hers.

"Uncle George, I can see by the twinkle in your eye that you're going to ask to kiss the bride," John noted amiably. "You may."

"Thanks, John. How'd you know?" Uncle George gave Mary a kiss on the cheek. "I must say I admire your taste. Prettiest bride I ever saw! Except one," he added quickly, with a sly glance at Aunt Emma.

"Come on in," Aunt Emma told them, ignoring his banter as she led them into the house. "You must be tired, and supper's ready and waiting. This will be your room, if you'd like to freshen up a bit." She opened the door to the guest room—really their own bedroom, but she and George were going to sleep on the porch that night so their young guests could have the only bedroom.

"You shouldn't do this," John chided her. "Mary and I can just as well sleep on the porch."

"Never argue with a woman, son," Uncle George advised. "I learned that long ago. Now whenever Em 'n' I have a disagreement I always have the last word, because to everything she says I reply, 'Yes, dear!' and that settles it!"

"Okay, Uncle George," laughed John. "C'mon, honey," he called to Mary, "we can bring our bags in here."

Supper was a simple one. Aunt Emma had fixed cold chicken and fruit, not knowing when the young folks would arrive. But she popped biscuits into the oven as soon as they came so there would be something hot.

"Are you still working in the lumberyard during summers?" Uncle George asked, stirring the third spoonful of sugar into his coffee.

"Yes," John replied. "I enjoy the outdoor work. It's a refreshing change from the classroom all winter, although I like teaching more than I thought I would. The best thing about my teaching is that it's in Pinedale. If I'd gone to some other school I might never have met Mary!" He smiled at her across the table. "By the way, Mary's quite a poet. You ought to hear some of the things she's written."

"May we, Mary?" asked Aunt Emma politely.

Mary blushed. "I'd—rather not, now. John is always bragging about me."

"Writing poems is nothing to be ashamed of, Mary," Uncle George told her gently. "I rather like to try my hand at it sometimes too. Em, where is that piece I wrote about the creation of the craggy cliff?"

"I think it's in the desk, George, in the lower left-hand drawer. Or maybe in that box of photos and clippings in the bedroom. Just a minute, I'll go see." Aunt Emma excused herself, returning a few minutes later with a yellowed paper. "Now wait a minute before you read it till I can bring out the pie and more hot coffee."

After everyone had been served dessert, Uncle George held his poem up to the lamp, cleared his throat, and read, in a voice almost as craggy as the cliff—

> Thou relic of an ancient glory
> Tell me, O rock! What is your story?
> What sculptor formed your stately ridge
> And chiseled it in arching bridge?
>
> Whose fingers moved to form thy face
> That time and tide cannot erase?
> Which ancient worker knew just how
> To hold his tools to shape your brow?

Who molded thy protruding chin
That stands so firm against the wind,
And planted trees upon thy shoulder?
O tell me this, thou time-worn boulder!

Who rounded out your stubby nose
And gave you rippling waves for clothes;
Who chiseled place for deep-set eye?
What was his name? Come! Make reply!

Then, as the breeze sighed through the pines,
I thought I heard him say these lines—
"The God who made earth, sky, and sea
Is He who also molded me."

"George reads his poems to people every chance he gets," commented Aunt Emma, "but I don't mind. Fact is, I enjoy them more each time I hear them."

"This one fits right in with the sermon we heard last month about God being such a wonderful Creator," John remarked. "You want to tell them about it, Mary?"

Mary declined. "You make a much better preacher than I do, honey. You tell them."

"Now that's a good combination!" chuckled Uncle George. "We have a poet and a preacher in our family too. I'm the poet, and Em's been preachin' at me ever since we were married!"

Aunt Emma didn't seem to mind his joking. Mary helped her clear the table and do up the few dishes after supper before they rejoined the men.

The steady creaking of the porch swing attested its great age as John and Mary sat in it together later, in the warm, gray-dark of the summer evening.

"Your father always loved that swing when he was a little boy," Aunt Emma remarked to John. "Many's the night I sat there with him in my arms after Mother died, and talked and sang to him until he fell asleep."

"I know. Dad's told me, Aunt Em. I loved this swing when I was little too. It's amazing that it still holds together. Maybe one of these days it'll just fall apart all at once!"

They all laughed. Uncle George hitched his rocker a little so he could see the stars. "I courted your Aunt Em in that swing," he said, "and if it could talk, what stories it could tell!"

"I'd like to hear them," said Mary, and they all laughed again.

"The swing can't talk—good thing," he winked at Aunt Em, "but I can tell you a story someone told us when we were first married. It's about the two bears that should be in every marriage. Ever hear it?"

"I've heard about the *three* bears," Mary volunteered, "but not about two."

"Now it's this way," Uncle George explained. "When two people fall in love, they can't see any fault at all in the loved one. Either their lover seems perfect to them, or else what little faults they notice don't matter at all. But after they're married, they find they're both human, after all. Each of them does things a little differently from the other, since they weren't brought up in the same home environment, and little habits of the other person begin to annoy. Sometimes unhappiness and cross words creep in even before the honeymoon's over."

John and Mary had stopped swinging. Each was thinking sheepishly of the cross words that had passed between them that very morning.

"Now if the two bears become a part of the marriage, everything will be all right," Uncle George went on. "The first bear is this: 'Bear ye one another's burdens, and so fulfill the law of Christ.' You'll find that one in Galatians if you look," he added with a twinkle in his eyes. "This sharing of burdens should be done not only with big problems, but with little ones as well," he continued. "If the husband always tries to see things from his wife's point of view, and the wife from her husband's, it will help them share each other's burdens and will keep them from offending each other even in little things.

"The second bear is this—the one in Colossians—'Forbearing one another, and forgiving one another, . . . even as Christ forgave you.' Married love is to be a forgiving love—putting up with the little things in the other person that annoy, in a spirit of love, not of martyrdom."

John reached for Mary's hand and pressed it tightly within his own in the dark. "Bear and forbear. Thank you, Uncle George. We'll try to keep the two bears a real part of our marriage."

"Who did George say was the preacher in our family?" smiled Aunt Emma. "We should let these children go to bed, George. They've had a long day traveling."

"Good night, Aunt Em," said Mary softly, as she and John walked toward the door. "Good night, Uncle George."

Chapter 3

Let Me Count the Ways

. . . rejoice with the wife of thy youth . . . and
be thou ravished always with her love. Prov.
5:18, 19.

Mary was humming to herself as she dusted the last few pieces of furniture in their little home. The doorbell rang just as she entered the bedroom to pick up the curtains she was making to brighten up the kitchen. She hurried to the door.

"Why, Mother! I wasn't expecting you this morning. Come on in." She gave her mother a quick embrace.

"I hadn't expected to stop by, Mary." Mrs. Johnson set her handbag on the counter as she spoke. "I thought that since I was out shopping, I might as well drop by for a minute. We still miss you so much at home."

"I'm glad you came, Mother. I've been having so much trouble with these curtains. Isn't this pretty material?" Mary held up the colorful print. "I picked the brown and yellow because John likes these colors best. But they won't hang straight, no matter what I do!"

Mrs. Johnson picked up one of the basted curtains and looked it over with an experienced eye. "Mary, you haven't drawn the threads. These will have to be done over. Don't you remember how I've shown you how to draw a thread at each end so the curtain will hang by the straight of the goods?"

18

Mary let out a discouraged sigh. How many times had her mother had her rip things out and sew them over!

"Don't be discouraged, Mary." Mrs. Johnson picked up one of the curtains and carried it over to the table. "Would you hand me the scissors, please? I'll stay long enough to help you pull the threads and hem these up again."

They both sat down and worked on the curtains for several minutes, while Mrs. Johnson gave the latest news of Jo Lynn's many activities. "By the way, Mary," she asked, attempting to sound offhand, "how are you and John getting along?"

"Just fine, Mother. And Mother, I'm so glad now for the things you taught me in high school." Mary absently let her curtain fall into her lap,—"Such as keeping my body as pure and new as my wedding dress. I wouldn't have thought of wearing my wedding dress before the day of the wedding. Now I'm so glad I kept myself for John too. You reminded me of the song that says

> Some day my Prince will come,—
> Some day I'll find my Love—

I had a lot of fun with the other kids at school, but none ever seemed so special as John."

"I'm glad for you, Mary," her mother said quietly, reaching for a thread and needle. "I believe that God has planned one special person for each of us, if it is His will for us to be married." She hemmed with neat, firm stitches as she spoke. "Married love has an especially deep meaning to those who have kept themselves true to just that one special person."

Mrs. Johnson hesitated. She wanted to say more but did not like to pry into the privacy of John and Mary's lives. "Mary, this hem is fixed, and I really must go now." She laid down the finished curtain. "Just one more thing I'd like to say—if you have any problems at all with the physical adjustments of marriage, don't hesitate to go back to Dr. Gordon for advice."

"We won't, Mother, although we really don't need to now. He gave us such helpful advice when we went to him before our marriage. Thanks so much for sending us to him!" She gave her mother a kiss and a wave as she went out the door.

After her mother had gone, Mary picked up the curtain and bent over her work again. Her cheeks flushed a little as she thought back to the conversation she and John had had with Dr. Gordon, and of how much it had helped them to find pleasure in their physical relationships.

"I assume that you young people are familiar with the physiology of the male and female," Dr. Gordon had said. "This information is now taught in the biology and family courses in many high schools and colleges. You know how the male glands secrete a solution called semen, in which are contained the tiny sperm that fertilize the egg of the female? When intercourse takes place, the male's penis—which becomes hard and erect when excited, ejaculates semen into the vagina of the female. When the ovum, or egg, of the woman is present at this time, the sperm fertilizes it and a new life begins to grow. You are familiar with this information?"

Both John and Mary nodded, so Dr. Gordon went on. "Now it has been assumed by some people that when God created us 'male and female' it was only for one purpose—the procreation of children, and that the pleasure and excitement of mating had no other justification. But if this is true, why is it that we're made so that the sexual urge doesn't disappear when childbearing age is past? We know, and the Bible teaches, that the act of mating is one that God planned in every detail, and which He meant to be a beautiful experience for the two people involved. The New Testament has some sound ideas on this. Remember the passage in Hebrews?" He reached for the Bible on the bottom shelf of his bookcase. "Here it is—Hebrews 13:4— 'Marriage is honourable in all, and the bed undefiled.' Corinthians is even more specific." The doctor turned the pages back to the passage. "Listen to this— 'Defraud ye not one the other, except it be with consent for a time, that ye may give yourselves to fasting and prayer; and come together again.' What Paul is saying is that neither the husband nor the wife has the right to avoid having intercourse with each other, unless they mutually agree to abstain during a specific period of prayer and fasting from food also. The wife is not to withhold her body from her husband, nor does the husband have the right to withhold his body from her. Each belongs to the other.

"In Ephesians 5 we even read that the sexual relationship between a man and his wife is a symbol of the relationship between Christ and the Church. 'This is a great mystery!' Paul says. The sexual relationship, of course, is itself a symbol of the 'oneness' of the marriage. Marriage is an institution created by God in which each partner is 'one' with the other all the time as well as during the sexual act, hurting or helping the other in everything each one does.

"In the Old Testament, too, we read of the beauty of the marriage relationship, especially in the Song of Solomon, which describes in allegorical form the physical pleasures of marriage. And in the Talmud it says that a Jewish wife even had the right to demand that her husband perform his sexual obligations to her!

"So we know that as an ideal the intercourse of marriage is holy and right in God's sight and that it's intended to be a delight for both husband and wife. The question in your minds just now, and in that of most young couples, about to be or just recently married, is how to make this ideal a reality in your own experience.

"Love-making can be satisfactorily fulfilled only where there is complete trust in each other, which is possible only in marriage. Yet it is such a revelation of the 'self' that even in marriage either partner can be deeply hurt by being casually 'used' by the other only for 'self'-satisfaction. Only where there is complete trust can love-making become such a delightful abandon of two persons to each other that they are as 'one,' body, soul, and spirit.

"When this trust and abandon is present, the mechanics of intercourse and its climax for both the man and the woman become the marvel that God's creative genius intended. For each of the pair, the climax consists of involuntary, rhythmical contractions. It is imperative that man be able to reach this climax so that he can send his fertilizing semen into the woman, or the human race would not survive. But because a woman can become pregnant without reaching this climax, it has often been assumed that the pleasure of sex was meant only for the male."

"I know that isn't true, doctor," John interrupted, "but the guys I know—" he paused, blushing slightly, "these guys say the girls never do reach a climax. I want Mary to be able to."

"Are these 'guys' married, John?" the doctor asked.

"Well, no, but I know some married guys who make the same complaint."

Doctor Gordon smiled. "Remember what I said about the ability to 'abandon' oneself in absolute trust to the other? This is not possible outside marriage. Both partners are cheated, and the man's mechanical orgasm is a poor substitute for the rich experience God intended. For a young woman, even after marriage her natural modesty is not overcome all at once as soon as the wedding is over. Her husband mustn't take advantage of her, simply because it is now legal to do so. He should respect her feelings of reserve and treat her gently, even though he may feel impatient.

"Further, although the sexual act may be completely satisfying to the husband, for his wife it is only the first step in the sexual cycle. She may not experience the fully mature response that God designed until after she's successfully completed the whole sexual cycle of intercourse, a healthy pregnancy, a happy natural birth experience, and pleasurable breast-feeding. The successful completion of this sexual cycle in a happy manner will give her a self-confidence, poise, and inner satisfaction with being a *woman* that she hasn't known before. She'll be able to abandon herself more freely to her husband and will consequently achieve a climax more easily. She will not be inhibited about skin-to-skin contact with her husband, any more than she is inhibited by the skin-to-skin contact of her nursing baby fondling her breast as he sucks contentedly. A woman must learn to *give* herself, if she is to be fully a woman.

"But let me go back now to the mechanics of sexual orgasm, which for both consists of a series of involuntary rhythmical contractions of a ring of muscular tissue. Much of life is rhythmical in similar ways. Our lungs expand and contract rhythmically as we breathe. Our heart and blood vessels rhythmically expand and contract. At the height of the male orgasm the ring of muscular tissue at the base of the erect penis contracts involuntarily and rhythmically to propel the semen as far as possible into the vagina of the woman. And at the height of female orgasm, the ring of muscular tissue *deep inside* the vagina involuntarily contracts rhythmically around the penis of her husband, sending waves of pleasure diffusing through her entire body.

"The basic difference in the sexual responses of the man and the woman is that the husband's desire is aroused more quickly and fades more quickly once orgasm is reached. The woman's desire is not only more slowly aroused, but once she reaches orgasm these involuntary vaginal contractions may recede, and then recur again and again several times over a period of twenty minutes or more. The involuntary contraction of the vaginal muscle stimulates contractions of the uterus as well until her whole being is caught up in the pleasure of this rhythm. Even her breathing rhythm may add to the total pleasure.

"This is the mature female orgasm, and it recedes slowly. The husband must continue to give her his attention and affection until it begins to fade, revealing how much he is interested in *her*, and not just in his own pleasure."

"But, doctor," Mary observed soberly, "are you saying that I won't be able to enjoy a climax until we've been married for years?"

"Not at all," the doctor laughed. "But you can reach this goal much more quickly by observing and practicing a few simple rules. The first one is to learn to contract your vaginal muscles *voluntarily*."

Mary frowned. "What do you mean? I thought you said the climax consisted of *in*voluntary vaginal contractions."

"It does. But if you learn to contract and relax these muscles alternately at will, this helps to trigger the involuntary contractions that bring such pleasure in intercourse."

"How do I do that? I don't even know where these muscles are!"

Patiently the doctor explained. "The vaginal wall is capable of the tremendous expansion necessary in the birth of a child. It is composed of layers of tissues drawn up tightly into folds by muscle fibers. The sphincter muscle that keeps the vagina closed is directly attached to the muscles that close the anus and the urethra. When one contracts, all three outlets contract. When one relaxes, all three relax. These muscles help form the 'floor' between the legs that give added support to the internal organs. If you cannot feel where these muscles are, cough.

"When you cough sharply, you will feel these muscles push out. Now reverse this pushing out and tighten these muscles, drawing them up toward the inside of the body. Hold them tightly for a count of three, then relax them slowly. If you are not sure you have relaxed them enough, cough again.

"Do this until you have learned to 'feel' exactly where these muscles are, and can tighten them or relax them at will. To practice, tighten, relax, tighten, relax, in a slow, even rhythm, up to twenty times.

"In preparation for coitus or intercourse, John, you should realize that in a woman the areas of sexual response are more widely diffused than in the man. The areas that respond to caresses with sexual excitement are the breasts, the clitoris (the small appendage between the vulva, or lips, just above the vagina, which looks rather like a miniature penis), the vulva, and the vagina itself. It is important to enjoy a period of caresses and affection before insertion. This stimulates the glands at the base of the vagina to release secretion which moistens the entrance, making insertion of the penis easier.

"Notice for example in the Song of Solomon, the emphasis upon fondling the breasts as a means of arousing the desires of the young wife. The clitoris also is stimulated by caresses of the surrounding tissue, though it may be sensitive to too much direct handling. Clitoral stimulation leads to a type of orgasm that is pleasurable, but less womanly and fulfilling than the deep vaginal orgasm which should follow.

"When both husband and wife are ready, there are still two

things that may cause difficulty with the first attempts at pene-tration by the husband. In some women the hymen, which is the small membrane which covers the opening of the vagina in a virgin, may be so thick or resistant to penetration that this causes pain. For this reason it should be gently dilated with the fingers first, and if it doesn't respond after five or six attempts at inter-course, it should be treated by a physician. In other girls, however, the hymen may be quite fragile and easily broken. It may already have been broken during some childhood accident.

"The second thing that may cause difficulty is a spasm of the vaginal muscles. One young wife said to me, 'But, doctor, I'm just too small for my husband!' Of course this wasn't true. What hap-pened was that this young bride was so fearful and anxious that she was not able to relax the sphincter muscle that closes the vagina. This resistance of the vaginal muscles is also an important cause of pain during childbirth. A woman *must* learn to relax these muscles at will.

"If she has not learned to do so before, it will help to open her mouth and inhale deeply, trying at the same time to 'let go' of the tension in the vaginal walls, and cough a time or two to help relax the outlet. The husband should then guide the penis carefully and gently so that it follows the slope of his wife's vagina and doesn't cause her discomfort. Often she can direct it herself so that it's comfortable for her.

"The insertion of the penis into the vagina is not the climax of intercourse, although this may cause such excitement to the young husband that it precipitates the climax for him. This may be dis-appointing to them both unless they realize that this is an experience to learn together, and that a sense of humor and a deep affection for each other will overcome all obstacles as time passes. One does not become a concert musician the first time he touches an instru-ment, nor can two beginning musicians play in absolute harmony. Time and experience, patience and humor will make the love-making more harmonious, more fulfilling, as time goes on. And even at the start, it can be fun!

"Once the penis is inserted about halfway, the husband should let it lie perfectly quiet. The walls of the vagina have few nerve endings, so that a rapid back and forth movement will only bring on a rapid climax for him, and not give pleasure to the wife. Immediately in back of the vaginal walls, however, are tissues with many nerve endings which respond pleasurably to *pressure* on the sides of the vagina. As the husband lies quietly, the wife should begin to consciously contract and relax the vaginal muscle rhythmically around her husband's penis. This adds to the pleasurable pressure in the vagina without overstimulating the husband. As she consciously contracts and relaxes this muscle and pleasure increases, before long the muscle of its own accord will involuntarily begin to do so, and she will have reached the threshold of orgasm. At this time the husband may begin to move the penis *slowly*, back and forth, pressing firmly against the vaginal walls as he does so, until his climax occurs. And when it does, he must be careful to continue showing his wife affection, until her own excitement begins receding.

"Keep in mind that the real goal is not just to come together to reach a climax, for this is only one small though important part of the total experience. The real goal is to enjoy each other throughout the entire love-making and give each other pleasure. To focus on the climax only is to inhibit its occurring properly and to miss much of the other joy that rightfully accompanies this whole experience."

The doctor paused, as if weighing over what he had said, and then added, "One other thing. John, there are some men who only show affection and caress their wives when they want coitus. If this is true of you, Mary may soon become resentful, and sex will lose its true meaning for you both. The subtle meaning behind every hug and kiss then becomes for her a signal that you want your sex hunger satisfied, rather than a sign that you really love *her*. The ability to show affection, hugging and kissing one's wife and children, makes a man a better husband and a better father, so that his children learn from the time they are small how to convey affection through cuddling and touch, and his wife feels secure in his love. You do want children, don't you?"

"Oh, yes!" Mary said quickly. "John and I have already talked about having children. Since he's through with his education, we won't need to use birth control. What do you think about birth control, doctor?"

"It's a very fine thing, Mary, when properly used in order to give a young couple time to adjust to each other after marriage before assuming family responsibilities, when used to conserve a young mother's energy, or in order to make sure the family can support the children they bring into the world. However, I believe that any means used for birth control is wrong when it's employed for purely selfish reasons—to avoid the trouble and expense of raising children."

"What about overpopulation?" John asked. "From all one hears about it, sometimes I wonder if it's right to have children at all!"

"The world wouldn't last long if that were true," the doctor smiled. "My personal belief is that this is a matter between a married couple and their God. Only He knows what children He wants born into their home, which particular children are to be born into which home. I do not believe this is a matter to be dictated by a government or even by a social code that says a man may have so many and no more. Since we know how to prevent conception, we already are able to prevent having a limitless number of children who cannot either be fed or clothed. But God may guide some parents to have five or six children and others to have only one. This is an intensely personal matter, and God's guidance will not be the same for each couple.

"What form of birth control do you recommend, doctor," John queried, "if we ever decide not to have any more children?"

"First, let me describe briefly several methods, and then I'll suggest what I think might be best for you, although it is really up to you.

"The first and oldest form of contraception (birth control is really 'conception' control) is simply abstinence—not having intercourse at all. Although certain religious elements in our society have objected to coitus except for the purpose of having children, abstinence is neither scriptural nor advisable, except for short periods of time under special circumstances, as we discussed earlier.

"The second simple and old form is 'coitus interruptus,' withdrawal of the penis before ejaculation. This is most unsatisfactory for both husband and wife, and she may become pregnant anyway, if a few sperm had escaped earlier.

"The condom—a thin rubber sheath that is pulled over the husband's erect penis—is simple and inexpensive, but it does detract a little from the pleasurable sensations involved, for there is not the sensitivity of skin-to-skin contact.

"The wife can be fitted by a doctor with a diaphragm, a rubber cup-shaped protection that she inserts into the vagina over the cervix, or mouth of the womb, prior to intercourse. The diaphragm must be used in combination with a spermacide (sperm-killing) cream, to be completely effective. The diaphragm is a bit of a nuisance to have to stop and insert before love-making, but it is highly effective, and does not in any way prevent the pleasure of the act.

"There are certain intrauterine devices that can be placed by the doctor which prevent the egg from imbedding itself in the wall of the uterus. This device stays in place until the doctor removes it. Occasionally, it slips out of place without the woman being aware of it, or, in some women, there may be some irritation within the uterus due to the presence of a foreign object."

"Why couldn't I just take birth control pills?" Mary wanted to know. "I have a lot of friends who do, and they say it's really easy. They don't have to worry about fooling with any of these other things."

"This may be the best solution for you, Mary, but there are a few other things to consider besides how 'easy' it is. We still do not know what the long-range effects of taking the pill might be, either on the woman herself, or on her children as they grow older. The pill also has potential health hazards for certain women, so that it should be prescribed for her only by a doctor well acquainted with her physical history. And there is one other problem. These same pills are used as 'fertility' pills to treat women who are infertile—that is, have difficulty becoming pregnant. After taking the pills a few months, it is stopped, and they seem to become pregnant much more readily. So a woman who decides to take the pill for a while, forgets to take them regularly as prescribed, or decides to quit after a while, actually is *more* likely to become pregnant than she was before starting the medication. Multiple births also occur more frequently to women who had been taking birth control pills earlier.

"My suggestion—unless for health or other serious reasons a woman should not risk a pregnancy at all—is to learn to use the sympto-thermal rhythm method. A woman is usually most fertile between the ninth and thirteenth day after the beginning of her menstrual cycle. During this fertile period intercourse can either be avoided, or else a condom or diaphragm used for a few days (either is preferable to a forced abstinence during this time).

"The fertility pattern of a woman is found in the Old Testament. She was considered 'unclean' for seven days following the end of menstruation, after which her husband could again have sexual union with her. The result of this law was to provide a very effective means of keeping the nation's population under control. Do you remember the story of David and Bathsheba in 2 Samuel 11? David saw her carrying out the washing ritual during the days following her period, sent for her, and lay with her without observing the seven days. She immediately conceived—of course!—much to his dismay.

"The problem with this method is that no two women have exactly the same fertile period, and even for the same woman it may vary a few days from month to month. There are two ways in which she can learn to recognize her fertile period, in addition to counting the days after menstruation begins. One symptom is that there is a slight temperature rise when she is fertile. She can check her temperature immediately upon awakening in the morning, either orally or rectally. After doing this a few mornings after each menstrual period for a few months, she will know on which days she is most likely to be fertile.

"The second way to tell is by the 'white loss,' a small discharge of stringy, stretchy white material from the vagina which shows that the unfertilized egg had left the womb. During the days of either temperature rise or white loss, some form of birth control should be used. Once the white loss has occurred, conception is not possible.

"Conversely, if there is difficulty in *becoming* pregnant, the couple should have intercourse on the days when this fertility is evident."

The doctor was silent, waiting for further questions, and leaned back in his chair. But he sat up abruptly when John said, "What about abortion? Isn't that a form of birth control, too?"

"Oh, my no!" the doctor exclaimed. "Abortion is an entirely different matter and must not be confused with the control of conception. You see, birth control *prevents* conception from taking place at all. Abortion, on the other hand, kills a living organism, the fetus whose life has already begun. I am not in favor of widespread abortion for any reason and certainly not as a means of population control.

"This is another big subject, and we can't go into it today. But let me show you one Scripture passage that reveals how important a subject this is. You see, many say that abortion on demand should be available when a woman and her doctor agree to destroy the living fetus. But the Bible says that this is a matter in which someone else is involved—the God who formed that child in the womb and who alone knows for what purpose that child is to live." Doctor Gordon reached across the desk for his Bible and opened it to Psalm 139 RSV:

> For Thou didst form my inward parts,
>   Thou didst knit me together in my mother's womb.
> I praise Thee, for Thou art fearful and wonderful.
>   Wonderful are Thy works!
>
> Thou knowest me right well;
>   My frame was not hidden from Thee
> When I was being made in secret,
>   Intricately wrought in the depths of the earth.

Thy eyes beheld my unformed substance;
  In Thy book were written, every one of them,
The days that were formed for me,
  When as yet there was none of them. . . .

"That's a sobering thought! Thank you, Dr. Gordon, so much," John said as the doctor rose, indicating that the interview was over. "This has all been most helpful."

"The best of happiness to you both," he smiled in response. "Don't hesitate to come in again if you have any problems."

"We certainly won't. Good-bye now."

The gay, new curtains were swinging merrily back and forth in the warm summer breeze swishing its way through the open window as Mary hurried to put the finishing touches on the pizza. Pizza was one of John's favorite dishes, and she hoped to have it ready when he came home from the lumberyard. As she heard the car door slam, she popped the pizza into the oven and set the timer for fifteen minutes—just long enough for John to get washed up for supper. A moment later he opened the door.

"Hi, honey! M-m-m-m! That pizza smells good!" He swept her into one arm, but kept the other behind him while he gave her a long kiss.

"John, what is that in your hand?"

"Guess."

"I can't. Tell me."

"It's a present for you, honey. Here. Open it." He handed her a small, flat package.

It had obviously been gift-wrapped in a store. Mary was sure that John couldn't tie a bow like that! She carefully untied the gold ribbon. She could feel the shape of a book beneath the flowered paper, and as she lifted it out John explained, "I stopped by the bookstore on the way home, Mary. I know how much you like the poems of Elizabeth Barrett Browning, so I got a copy of them for you. I've picked one out to read you. Listen."

He opened the book to a place he had marked, and slipped his arm around her waist. Mary laid her head on his shoulder as he read—not minding at all that he smelled of sawdust and the sweat of honest labor—

How do I love thee? Let me count the ways.
I love thee to the depth and breadth and height
My soul can reach, when feeling out of sight
For the ends of Being and Ideal Grace.
I love thee to the level of every day's
Most quiet need, by sun and candlelight,
I love thee freely, as men strive for Right;
I love thee purely, as they turn from Praise;
I love thee with the passion put to use
In my old griefs, and with my childhood's faith.
I love thee with a love I seemed to lose
With my lost saints,—I love thee with the breadth,
Smiles, tears of all my life!—and, if God choose,
I shall but love thee better after death.

Chapter 4

My Father's World

*The earth is the Lord's, and the fulness
thereof; the world, and they that dwell
therein.* Ps. 24:1.

The golden warmth of the September sun flooding the landscape
was reflected in the brilliant gold, orange, and scarlet foliage of
the woodland trees, framed as they were against the dark green
shades of the evergreens. The Johnsons and the Thomases were
taking advantage of the sunny Saturday for a late drive along the
river.

"We must be almost to the bridge," Jo Lynn remarked, leaning
forward and tipping her head a little to see out of the windshield
past her mother in the front seat.

"It won't be long now, Jo Lynn," her father answered. "The
scenery along here is so colorful that it would be a shame to
hurry by."

"How much farther is it to the falls after we reach the bridge?"
John asked.

"Not very far. I've forgotten exactly," Mr. Johnson replied.
"Here's the bridge now." He slowed the car and turned it toward the
bridge approach.

"Wow! This is some bridge!" John exclaimed. "We seem to be
a mile above the river!"

33

The teal-blue splendor of the magnificent river far below them stretched in both directions as far as they could see. On their left, its broad expanse plunged toward them through the channel it was forging in the mountains; on their right, its turbulent water churned onward in its restless quest for oblivion within the bosom of the ocean.

As they turned west onto the river highway, they could see, back on the other side, the scenic road that they had just left, drawn like a curved white chalk line through the green and orange foliage along the north banks of the river. After only a few moments on the highway they arrived at the falls.

"Here we are!" cried Jo Lynn, preparing to hop out of the car the minute her father parked it in the lot near the falls.

"Let's take our lunch to those tables up near the little bridge over the falls," Mrs. Johnson suggested, as they all piled out of the car. "Jo Lynn! Come back here and help carry some of these things." Jo Lynn came back reluctantly, and took a box to carry. With everyone helping, they soon had the lunch deposited on the picnic table.

"I'll stay at the table," Mrs. Johnson offered, "so you youngsters and Dad can hike the rest of the way to the top of the falls."

Mrs. Johnson opened one of the boxes and began spreading out the picnic cloth. Jo Lynn was already bounding up the mountainside, her dad right behind her, John and Mary close on his heels. The falls loomed above them, a spectacular drop to the river far below.

"John!" Mary gasped. "Please stop."

"Why, honey, what's the matter? Here, sit on this rock a minute." He drew her to the side of the path and set her on a small boulder.

"I—don't know." Mary felt very faint, and leaned against him until she could focus her eyes more clearly. "I guess—we were going up too fast. I never felt this way before!—I'm better now. Let's go on." She stood up, but John eased her gently back onto the rock.

"What's the matter, Mary?" her dad asked. He and Jo Lynn

came back toward them. "Were we setting too fast a pace? You look pale."

"I'm all right now. Let's go on up." Mary got up, but Mr. Johnson took her arm and turned her toward the descent.

"Look, Mary. Let's you and I go back and help Mother set out the lunch. John and Jo Lynn can go on up to the top of the falls. I've been there many times before, but John ought to see it."

Mary consented reluctantly. Jo Lynn gaily took John's arm, swung around flippantly, and looked back at Mary with a broad, teasing wink. Mary made a face at her behind John's back. Usually she didn't mind Jo Lynn's joking, but this time she felt unaccountably irritated.

"Don't mind her, Mary." Her father patted her arm. "John wouldn't look at her twice if they were marooned on a desert island."

"I know that, Dad. It's just that . . ." Mary's sentence trailed off unfinished, as they walked leisurely back down the trail. Mary loved her dad and the way he understood so many things about her without her having to explain.

Mrs. Johnson looked up in surprise when she saw them coming. After observing her daughter's behavior unobtrusively for a moment, she quietly drew her own conclusions.

"There's something that has always bothered me," John remarked thoughtfully. They had parked in one of the places provided along the highway on their way home, and were walking over to sit on the stone ledge overlooking the river. "I've been thinking about it all day. I've been so conscious today of God's presence in the world as I've seen the splendor of this area. But, since He is present in our world, *why* is there so much suffering?"

"That's a hard question," Mr. Johnson answered. He paused a moment, looking around him, and then said, "Mother, come sit over by me. You can see better here, and the wall's a little smoother to sit on." After seeing that she was comfortable, he returned to John's question. "Ever since the time of Job people have pondered over the problem of pain, and there are no easy answers."

"Some people say that all suffering is the result of sin," Jo Lynn interrupted, "but I don't see how that could be. When that little girl in the next block was hit by a car, was it because she was so evil? And is old Mrs. Arkwright all crippled up with arthritis because she didn't live right? It doesn't make sense to me."

"Some suffering is certainly the result of sin, Jo Lynn," her father answered. "Sin has marred the perfect artistry of God, and countless numbers have died beneath bombs that man has made from the knowledge God has given us that we've corrupted. You see, God has given man a *free will*, and with this freedom of choice comes the peril of man not going the right way, God's way. Such a man leaves a trail of suffering in his path of evil doing. For example, perhaps the fellow who ran over little Laurie was exceeding a safe speed limit or had been drinking. Ignoring the welfare of other people is certainly sin. But this makes the problem harder— often people suffer not because of their *own* sin, but because of the sins of other people."

"To say that all suffering is the result of sin is too simple an answer then, isn't it?" Mary asked. "But the Jews of Jesus' day seemed to believe this. Remember, Dad, when they asked Him about the blind man, 'Who did sin, this man, or his parents, that he was born blind?' and Jesus answered, 'Neither hath this man sinned, nor his parents.' "

"That's right, Mary," her father agreed. "So there must be additional causes for suffering. There is also what we call the 'accidents of nature.' God has set up certain unchanging physical laws that govern the universe, and these laws operate without discrimination. Jesus said of the Heavenly Father, 'He maketh his sun to rise on the evil and on the good, and sendeth rain on the just and on the unjust.'

"The small child who falls into a river and drowns is an illustration of this. It wouldn't make any difference if the child was good or bad, a boy or a girl, English or Chinese, Hindu or Christian. The unchanging chemical formula of the water would cause its death. But what would happen if this formula for water was constantly changing? Human life couldn't survive if the balance of hydrogen and oxygen in water wasn't a stable one."

"But then, Dad," Mary said, "wouldn't it be all right to say that suffering either from sin, or from an accident of nature, is caused by an interference with the harmony of God's natural law?"

"I'm inclined to agree with you, Mary," John spoke up. "So much suffering is caused by ignorance, as in places where nutrition and sanitation aren't understood. This destroys the harmony of God's laws too—but surely He didn't intend for people to be ignorant of the simple laws of the natural world He created, did He?"

"I'm sure He didn't," Mr. Johnson replied. "Some have called this breakdown in the harmony of His laws the theory of a disordered universe, due to the presence of evil forces in the world. The Bible teaches that there is a source of evil which existed even before man, and that if it weren't for God's staying hand, the whole universe would be in chaos.

"Jesus identifies this source of evil as 'Satan,' and says that Satan is responsible for much of the ignorance, sickness, and tragedy present in the world. For example, when Jesus saw the woman who had been crippled for eighteen years, He said, 'Ought not this woman . . . whom Satan hath bound' to be made well? And He healed her."

"This is the comforting thing to remember," Mrs. Johnson added, speaking up for the first time as they walked slowly back to the car, "that no matter what may have caused the suffering, God can bring peace of mind, and restoration to health, or strength to bear the trial graciously." After they had settled into their places and driven back out onto the highway, she went on, "I've been so impressed in reading Mark again, with Jesus' concern for the sick. Everywhere He went He not only taught the people, but He also healed them. He didn't heal everyone in Palestine, but He did heal all those who came to Him."

"Yes," Mr. Johnson concluded. "Jesus is revealed in the Gospels as being concerned for the whole man—body, mind, and spirit. Remember, too, that He taught that God is our Heavenly Father, concerned with every need of ours. The New Testament says over a hundred and fifty times that God is our Father."

"That reminds me of the song we used to sing when I was a boy,"

John reminisced, "called 'This Is My Father's World.' I haven't thought of it in a long time. I like the part that says that

> Though the wrong seems oft so strong,
> God is the Ruler yet!"

They had recrossed the bridge and were winding quickly along the twisting road on the other side of the river.

"Dad, aren't you going awfully fast?" Mary finally asked. She had tried to endure the lurching in the back seat as long as she could but was getting sicker by the minute. "I think you'd better stop!" she warned.

Mr. Johnson pulled off to the side of the road, and helped her from the car. "You and Mother trade places, Mary," he told her, "and you can sit up in front with me where the riding's smoother."

"On second thought," he added, after glancing into the back seat and noticing the mischievous look on Jo Lynn's face, "why don't you drive, John? I haven't had a chance to sit in the back and hold hands with Mother for a good many years!"

Chapter 5

Tinier Than a Raindrop

As thou knowest not what is the way of the spirit, nor how the bones do grow in the womb of her that is with child; even so thou knowest not the works of God who maketh all. . . . Lift up your eyes on high, and behold who hath created these things. . . .
Eccles. 11:5, Isa. 40:26.

Mary gazed out the window of the doctor's waiting room at the gentle balm of rain. I can't understand why some people feel that the rain is depressing, she thought to herself. So many times as a little girl I lifted my face to feel the raindrops, and thought how good God was to me. And now I'm so happy! To think that there's a new life growing in my body seems like a dream—a new life that was tinier than a raindrop at first! I know God's love is within me, all around me, enveloping the whole world as the rain refreshes the thirsty earth. Oh, how I love Him! And everybody!

Mary glanced around the room. What a pretty outfit, she thought, a bit covetously, noticing the woman sitting just opposite her. I wonder how far along she is. She looks pretty big—maybe her baby is about due. I can hardly wait to go shopping for my outfits. Won't Joanie be jealous! They've been married two years now. Of course, it would be fun to keep it a secret as long as we could—she glanced over at John, buried in a magazine—but it's so exciting I just *have* to tell somebody. What a darling little girl that is walking by outside with the pink umbrella! I wonder if we'll have a girl, or a boy. We'll have to think about names—

"Mr. and Mrs. Thomas, will you step in now, please?" The nurse's voice broke into Mary's reverie. John laid down his magazine, and he and Mary followed the nurse down the hall to Dr. Gordon's office.

"Hello! Come on in," Dr. Gordon greeted them warmly. "How's the teaching this year, John? I've noticed the team's doing very well this fall." He motioned to the chairs near his desk, and John and Mary sat down.

"It's going pretty well," John replied. "I don't have as many problem youngsters in my history classes, and, of course, we're all happy about the performance of the team. The boys are taking their training rules seriously this year, and it sure makes a big difference in their game!"

"I'm hoping to get to tomorrow night's game, but don't count on it." Dr. Gordon had seated himself behind his desk. "What can I do for you young people today? You're not having any problems, I trust?"

"No, it's just that—" Mary blushed slightly, "I think we're going to have a baby."

"That's good news. Can you tell me what makes you think so?"

"Well," Mary answered, twisting her purse handle around her fingers as she spoke, "I've missed my last two periods, and this has never happened to me before. Also, I've noticed that my breasts are a bit larger."

Dr. Gordon nodded. "These are good indications of pregnancy. Other signs may include more frequent urinating, as the growing uterus presses against the bladder, or slight skin changes. Sometimes fatigue and nausea occur. Have you had any problem with either, Mary?"

"No," she said, thinking back, "except for one time when we went to the falls with my folks. I was rather miserable part of the time, but then we did quite a little hiking, and Dad drove home pretty fast."

"Nature puts out little warning signs when we're doing too much," Dr. Gordon smiled. "A girl who's carrying a child soon learns that she'll have to make a few adjustments, and take things at a more leisurely pace. Real fatigue in pregnancy, though, if one is not overactive, may be a sign of poor nutrition, or it may indicate that inwardly the mother is a little unhappy over being pregnant. We're learning more all the time about the important relationship between the state of a person's mind and the functioning of his body.

"The same thing is true of nausea. Occasionally, the glandular changes that take place when pregnancy begins cause disturbances of other functions, but many women have no difficulty with this at all. Frequently, when nausea persists, I suspect that there are other problems creating tensions, which show up in this way, as well as in fatigue. Sometimes there are financial or marital difficulties that the mother is worried about, or she may be anxious because this is a new and untried experience for her.

"Learning to relax helps to relieve nausea if it has been caused by tension or worry. Eating small meals frequently rather than three large ones, or munching crackers between meals helps. Sometimes a light breakfast in bed before getting up will prevent discomfort in the morning."

"I get the hint!" John grinned. "Now don't start pretending to have nausea, Mary, so you can have breakfast in bed!"

"Not a bad idea," Mary laughed, "and how could you tell if I *was* pretending?"

"Perhaps we'd better change the subject," Dr. Gordon suggested, smiling, "before I get involved in a family controversy! By the way, Mary, next month we'll give you a complete physical examination to be sure everything is progressing normally. As a rule, I like to use the first prenatal visit to get acquainted and put the expectant parents at ease, but that's hardly necessary in your case. Of course, if you had come in later in your pregnancy, or if there were any indications of any problem, we would go ahead immediately with a complete examination. But today you will get off lightly. The nurse will check your blood pressure, weight, and test a urine sample, and we'll do these three things each time you come in. We'll test your blood from time to time to be sure you're not anemic.

"I want you to call me at once if you notice any persistent headache, swelling or puffiness of your legs or other parts of your body, or any sudden weight gain, as these are danger signals and should be treated at once. Call me right away, too, if you have any vaginal bleeding.

"Avoid having intercourse during the time when your menstrual period normally occurs, as this might cause you to miscarry. Otherwise, normal intercourse is all right, if it is gentle, and not too frequent. It is usually wise to avoid intercourse during the last weeks of pregnancy.

"Now, the most important thing for you to learn, Mary, is to master the art of relaxation. Learning to relax during pregnancy will make it possible for your baby to be born without your needing sedation, or with very little. Not only will you have a happier, more comfortable labor this way, but it will be safer, too."

"That's something I've wanted to ask you about, doctor," Mary said soberly. "I've heard so many awful things about women suffering whenever a baby is born, but I just can't believe that it was meant to be that way. It doesn't fit with what I've always been taught about the Creator being a God of love. It seems to me that when He gives us a little baby it ought to be a really happy time— but even Mother won't talk about when Jo Lynn and I were born!"

"I'm glad you asked this, Mary," he answered her, in the same sober vein, "if it's troubled you. You see, we doctors have learned that babies can be born not only without a mother's suffering, but with great happiness for her, in the majority of cases. Even for the small percentage of mothers whose deliveries present difficulties, the ability to relax will make the needed medication more effective. I've changed from my former approach to obstetrics—and it takes a real struggle with our pride for us doctors to admit we've been wrong about anything, and to change our minds! But I feel so differently about obstetrics now that sometimes, Mary, when I remember how I delivered babies like you, I feel that I should apologize to your mothers!

"When the labor of childbirth begins, the muscles of the uterus, or womb, contract periodically, gradually and gently pushing the baby's head out of the uterus down into the 'birth canal.' This is the 'first stage' of labor. As the uterine muscles contract, they also shorten, drawing up the cervical muscles of the uterine outlet so that the baby can slip through easily.

"The uterine muscles are 'smooth' muscles, similar in structure and function to muscles of other internal organs that rhythmically contract and relax, such as the stomach, with few nerve endings. A normal uterine contraction causes no more pain than a normal stomach contraction. But, during labor, the tightening of these uterine muscles cause it to tilt forward against the muscles of the abdominal wall, and the baby begins to move downward against the muscles and tissues of the pelvic floor. When a woman feels the slight pressures from these changes of position, she becomes aware that labor has begun. Her *reaction* to this awareness determines whether or not she will begin to have pain.

"For the skeletal muscular tissues of the abdomen, back and pelvic floor are liberally supplied with sensory and pain receptors. If these muscles are contracted, in fear of the contracting uterus, pain is caused, not in the uterus itself, but *in all these surrounding tissues.* This is the so-called 'pain' of labor, and it really hurts! But if the surrounding muscular tissues remain relaxed and do not resist the uterus in its work, the cause for pain is absent. Thus a woman *creates her own pain* by inadvertently tightening her abdominal muscles and thus interfering with the normal work of the uterus.

"So you can see how important it is for a person to be able to 'let go' of muscle tension throughout the body for a comfortable birth. But muscular relaxation is also tremendously important for basic good health in all of life, so you should *both* learn it well.

"We hear a great deal these days about the 'stress' diseases, nervous indigestion, colitis, ulcers, headaches, backaches, high blood pressure, chronic fatigue, heart trouble. All of these things, in addition to pain in childbirth, are among the adverse effects of stress on the human body. We cannot get rid of stress in our environment, but we can learn to respond without an excess of muscular tension. Some people are so 'up tight' that they never relax their skeletal muscles properly, even in sleep!

"Relaxation is a condition in which muscle tone throughout the body is reduced to a minimum, and all the skeletal muscles are 'limp,' 'loose,' with as little tension as a cooked string of spaghetti or a wet noodle. Why waste muscle energy when we don't need it? We need to give serious thought to the advice of the wise aged black man who was asked how he'd managed to live so long. He said, 'Well, when ah works, ah works hard, but when ah sits, ah sits *loose!*'"

"This makes sense to me," John spoke up. "I think we live in an awfully tense, fidgety, restless way most of the time today. I try to explain to my athletes that if their muscles are tense all the time their co-ordination will be poor, and they're bound to fumble the ball a lot more. They have to learn when muscle tension is needed, and how to 'let go' the tension in those same muscles when the tension is not needed in order to play a good game."

"Exactly," the doctor said. "Now, Mary, I'm going to lift your hand to see how well you can relax. You are to let it *drop* onto the table. No, you're putting it down with your muscles, not letting it drop. Here," he took hold of her forearm again, "let me shake your arm so the hand flops like a leaf in the wind."

Patiently he worked with her until she was able to relax the muscles of her hand enough to let it drop limply. "Now," he said, laying her forearm on the table, her hand down, placing his finger across the back of her wrist, "lift one of your fingers, and tell me when you can feel which muscles are working."

"My finger muscles," Mary said.

"Do it very, very slowly, and tell me what muscles you feel working *before* you begin to lift your finger, as soon as you feel any tension at all."

"Why, I can feel the muscles pull on the back of my hand and up the forearm, even before I lift my finger!" Mary exclaimed.

"Exactly. Now let's do it again, and this time 'let go' this muscle tension just as soon as you begin to feel it, when you just *think* about raising your finger." Mary did so.

"I see what you're driving at, doctor," John said. "You want her to learn what tension *feels* like in every muscle, so she'll know when she's *not* relaxed."

"Right," the doctor agreed. Turning to Mary, he said, "I'm giving you these instructions on how to relax, Mary." He handed her a small folder. "The next time you come in I'll test you to see how well you've learned to do it. You can help her with this, John.

"In fact," he added, "it's my conviction that the husband has a most important role to perform throughout his wife's experience. You can help Mary in many ways, John, by encouraging her to learn proper relaxation, to follow my instructions about weight and exercises, and, most of all, by giving her your patient understanding. When it's time for the baby to be born, you can stay with her and help her throughout the labor and birth, if you wish. I'll show you what to do at that time to make it a wonderful experience for both of you."

"I'd like that very much," John said emphatically. "There are so many stories of the useless husband pacing the floor or reading a paper upside down, while his wife's in another room giving birth. It annoys me. I want to help Mary in every way I can."

"But how can we know when our baby's supposed to be born?" Mary asked. "Can you tell exactly when it will be?"

"Not exactly, Mary, but within a few days, either way. When was your last menstrual period?"

"Let's see." Mary thought a moment. "It was about July twentieth. I can check for sure when we get home."

"To arrive at the approximate date, think back three months and add seven days. That would be April twenty-seventh, wouldn't it?" He marked it down on her chart. "Do you have any other questions? If not, you may go into the laboratory now, Mary, so the nurse can check the things I've indicated.

"By the way," he called them back as they turned to go out the door, "why don't you ask Carolyn Thebes, Mary, about how her babies were born? She's had three beautiful natural births, and she can spend more time explaining how it should be than I can."

"I'll do that," Mary said. "Thank you for all the time you've given us already." Before following the nurse down the hall, she said to John, "You know who Carolyn is, don't you, dear? She's Paulie's mother."

"You're not really relaxed, Mary," John said to her that evening as she was trying it for the first time. "Your lips are twitching, and you keep shifting your left foot a little."

Mary was lying on her back on the floor, one pillow under her head and shoulders, and another large pillow under her knees. Her feet were about twelve inches apart with each foot falling outward. She was trying to lie as limply and loosely as a rag doll. When John spoke to her, she concentrated on her left foot a moment, tightened its muscles just a little, and then let it fall more limply outward than before. To relax her lips, she tightened them, and then let them fall slightly apart. She squeezed her eyes tighter, before letting the muscles of her eyelids and forehead become limp, too.

"Much better," John told her. "Now lie perfectly still—the folder says you shouldn't shift or move a muscle for thirty minutes. You've got twenty minutes to go. I'll tell you when time's up." He set his watch on the arm of the couch where he could see it and picked up the newspaper. Pulling the footstool toward him, he placed his feet on it, letting them fall limply outward in a relaxed manner, as Mary's were. He took a slow deep breath and then let the muscles of his abdomen and back relax, so that he slumped down comfortably against the back of the couch.

After lying down, Mary had begun relaxing by taking a deep breath, holding it for a count of five, and then letting it out slowly, slowly, slowly, letting her abdomen and chest wall collapse of its own weight limply as she exhaled. She had paused a second or two, then taken another deep breath, this time concentrating on letting her *abdomen* rise, rather than her chest, and again she had let her abdominal muscles become limper and limper as she let her breath out slowly. She continued breathing in this way several times after John spoke to her, each time letting all the joints and muscles of her entire body become more limp with each outgoing breath. Soon she was breathing deeply and evenly without needing to give it any more thought. Her arms and legs were beginning to prickle and seemed almost numb, as if they were becoming detached from her body, and she felt as if she were about to float off into space.

"Time's up," John said, when the thirty minutes had passed. "Get up slowly, so you won't get dizzy."

"There's nothing very hard about that!" Mary exclaimed, as she sat up. "I don't think I've ever been so completely relaxed in my whole life!"

"Remember that Dr. Gordon said you must do this *faithfully,*" John warned her. "I'm going to check up on you. You're supposed to learn to become completely limp within a minute or two after lying down."

"I wasn't very relaxed until a few minutes before you called time, John, but I don't think it'll take so long next time, now that I know how to do it. And I *intend* to practice faithfully, for my baby's sake especially."

"I'm all for you, honey," John encouraged her, as he drew her down onto the couch beside him. "Why don't we read through these instructions once more," he suggested, as he flipped the folder open again, "just to be sure we're doing this right."

RELAXATION

A. Learn to recognize tension.

There is no such thing as a relaxation "exercise," as the two are direct opposites. But follow the procedure below until you are *sure* you can recognize the difference between tension and relaxation in your own body.

Make your hand *slowly* into a fist, noticing what the muscles feel like as they tighten. Slowly, slowly, "let go" of the tension in the muscles of your hand, noticing at each step how it feels. When the hand seems completely limp, let it relax still more, and more, noticing carefully how it *feels* as it becomes completely relaxed. Repeat with the other hand, slowly making a fist, slowly relaxing the hand muscles, paying careful attention to how it feels at all stages.

Tighten the muscles of the right arm *slowly*, observing the "pull" of the muscles throughout the arm. Very slowly release the muscular tension. When the arm seems completely limp, relax it some more. Relax it still further.

Repeat this with the left arm, then with each foot and with each leg. Lift each leg *slowly*, noticing how it feels, then let it fall limply. Relax the muscles further. When it seems completely limp, "let go" the muscles still more. You will be surprised at how much tension is still there to "let go!"

Now tighten the muscles of your chest and shoulders, slowly, slowly, so you can feel each muscle pulling. Now slowly relax them, letting the shoulders droop and the chest collapse, continually noticing how different the muscles feel as they relax.

Tighten the muscles of your face and neck slowly, and frown. Slowly relax these muscles, thinking all the time of how it feels. When your face seems completely relaxed, relax your forehead and eyelids still more. Relax your neck slowly, until it droops forward on your chest, too limp to support your head.

Tighten the muscles of the pelvic floor (the area between the legs, including the anus, vagina, and urethra). Hold for a count of three, and then relax slowly, slowly, more and more, and more. Still more.

B. *Relax in the following manner each day.*
Empty the bladder before beginning, and remove all tight clothing —shoes, belts, collars, etc.

Lie on your back on a firm bed, or on a folded blanket on the floor, with one pillow under your head and shoulders, and another under your knees. It may be more comfortable to use one pillow under each knee. Roll the pillows so that the knees are supported four or five inches off the floor and are several inches apart. Rest the arms on the floor, with the elbows bent slightly outward. No part of the body should rest on any other, and every joint should be slightly bent.

Take a slow, relaxed breath deep into the chest and abdomen, and let it out slowly, relaxing the chest and abdominal wall as the air is released. Pause a moment before taking another breath, then breathe in slowly, breathe out slowly, in slowly, out slowly, relaxing the muscles more and more with each outgoing breath. This is called "sleep" breathing, the abdominal wall gently rising and falling as if you were asleep, and the breathing becoming slower and slower until it is barely noticeable.

Go limp all over as quickly as possible, letting all joints and limbs be as loose as if you were "falling through the floor."

Do not shift or move for thirty minutes, even to look at the time. Set an alarm, or have someone call when time is up.

Arms and legs will soon seem detached, as if "floating." They may have transient "pins and needles" as relaxation deepens.

When the time is up, get up slowly, to avoid dizziness.

Relax all muscles in this manner near the middle of each day. Do it again on going to bed. You will go to sleep quickly and will "sleep like a baby."

Chapter 6

The Joyful Mother of Children

*. . . happy shalt thou be, and it shall be well
with thee. . . . Thy wife shall be as a fruitful
vine by the sides of thine house: thy children like olive plants round about thy table.*
Ps. 128:2, 3.

"Why Mary! Come on in!" Carolyn greeted her warmly as she held
the door open. "I haven't seen you since the day of the wedding.
You look marvelous! And what a lovely outfit! This *is* a surprise."

"It does seem like a long time since I was here," Mary said,
when Carolyn stopped talking long enough for her to answer.
"Just think!" she said dreamily, "I was still Mary Johnson then. It
seems like years ago."

Carolyn drew up a chair for Mary near the table where she had
been working on a pile of mending. "You don't mind if I keep
sewing while we visit, do you?" she asked, picking up the button
jar and a small pair of torn overalls.

"Not at all," Mary answered. "Carolyn," she asked, after glancing around the room and noticing the sewing machine placed in
the middle of the playpen, "what in the world have you done *that*
for?"

Carolyn chuckled as she explained. "Baby Greg is always unhappy when I put him in there, but if I let him out, he and Julie
keep trying to climb onto my lap while I'm sewing, or stepping on

the machine pedal by mistake, so—I decided to put the machine where they couldn't reach it. Now they can play happily in the room, and I get into the playpen and sew in peace."

"It'd take a genius to think of a solution like that!" Mary teased her, "or a nut," she added slyly. "It seems so quiet here today. Is Paulie in school? It must be a help to have him out of the house part of the time."

"Paulie really enjoys kindergarten," Carolyn replied, "but Julie is so lonesome with just the baby, that I often wish he were still here to play with her. By the way, I'm terribly sorry about his dropping the ring at your wedding. I'd stitched it to the pillow with only one loop so it could be pulled off easily, but he must have picked at it beforehand so it fell off."

"Don't worry about that the least bit," Mary reassured her. "Thinking back on it now, it's even funny—he'd tried so hard to do everything just right, bless his heart."

"Let's hear the news about you, Mary," Carolyn suggested, reaching for another small pair of overalls to mend. "I didn't expect to see you in a maternity dress already."

Mary smiled. "Mother tried hard to convince me to wait longer before buying one, especially since we've been married such a short time—but I've been so happy and excited I've wanted everybody to know about our baby."

"That's an awfully pretty dress," Carolyn observed, "but you'll sure get tired of it before nine months are over. I've several smocks you can borrow—it's more fun to have several changes. Of course, everyone in Pinedale will know where you got them!"

"I don't mind if they do. That's kind of you, Carolyn." Mary hesitated a moment, and then said, "You know, this is one of the things I came to talk to you about today—I mean about having my baby. Dr. Gordon said I ought to come see you, as you'd had three natural births, and would have more time to explain things to me than he had."

"I'll be glad to help you. Ralph and I want to do all we can to help other couples have happy times when their babies are born, as we have. And this is a good time to talk while Julie and Greg are taking their naps." She glanced toward the bedroom door to reassure herself that they were still asleep, and then began telling Mary her own experiences.

"We waited eight years, Ralph and I, for our first baby. We both had tests of all kinds that showed that there was nothing wrong, but still we didn't have any success. We prayed about our problem, too, until finally I decided to stop fretting, and just relax and trust God. I thought of the verse in the Bible that says, 'He maketh the barren woman to keep house, and to be a joyful mother of children,' and I felt that if it was God's will for me, I would really be a mother some day—either to my own, or to someone else's homeless child.

"We had begun to apply to adoption agencies, when one day, we found that our dreams had come true. I began to experience what I had always felt in my heart—that carrying a baby and giving him birth is one of the most wonderful things that can happen to a woman. I wouldn't trade one moment of my experiences for anything in the world!"

"You certainly sound different from others I've heard," Mary commented wryly.

"That's because a lot of women don't understand a natural birth," Carolyn explained, "and they confuse it with stoicism—but it's really so exciting that after Paulie was born, I would have liked to have a baby every year! The only trouble with *that* is—it's too wearing running after too many little tots, when they're so close together.

"When I first became pregnant with Paulie, I went to an obstetrician of good reputation where Ralph was stationed. He did a routine examination but explained nothing to me. As I was going out, he patted my arm kindly and said, 'Cheer up, Mrs. Thebes. This is a sickness that only lasts for nine months!' Believe me, I never went back to him again! A *sickness,* of all things! To me it was a privilege to be pregnant, and I was very happy.

"Before long we moved to Pinedale, and I went to Dr. Gordon. I'll never forget his response when I told him I wanted to have a natural birth. He said, 'Carolyn, I'll do everything I know to help you have the kind of birth experience you want.'

"I asked him if Ralph could be with me during both my labor and the birth, and he said yes, 'your husband will be a big help to you.' Then I said I wanted to be propped up for the second stage of labor. He agreed to this, too. By this time I could hardly believe my ears, but I thought I might as well ask the rest, so I told him I wanted to hold my baby as soon as possible after he was born and breast-feed him if he wished. I certainly thought that would stop him, but it didn't. But he did warn me that I would have to prepare for a natural birth ahead of time, since it was not an experience that a woman in our culture can have just by wishing for it. Mary, you're really fortunate to have such an understanding and well-informed doctor. Be sure to do everything he tells you."

"I certainly will," Mary assured her soberly. "But Carolyn, can you tell me what happens when a baby is born? I mean, what does it actually *feel* like to have a baby without any sedatives or anesthetics?"

"It's this way," Carolyn explained patiently. "When labor first begins, the uterus, or womb, contracts rhythmically in order to push the baby gradually out through the cervix—the mouth of the womb—into the birth canal. This is called the first stage of labor, when the uterine muscles tighten, relax, tighten, relax. God planned it this way, so that the blood supply of these muscles would be constantly replenished, and so that pain would be avoided by having the uterine muscles alternately work and rest. The cervix is thinned out and stretched slowly, little by little, to allow the baby's head to be eased through it—rather the way one might stretch a rubber band to slip a ball through.

"During this period you have to relax all muscles *completely*. You see, you feel pain in labor whenever the muscles of the abdominal wall are kept tense while the uterus is rising during contractions. When a mother does this—usually without realizing she's doing it, the aching in these abdominal muscles increases with each contraction and soon spreads throughout the muscles of the pelvic area, making them ache, across the muscles of the lower back and hips, and even down into her thighs, so she literally 'aches all over' during the remainder of the labor, with increasing intensity. Each time a woman grips the railing of her bed as a contraction begins, and grits her teeth against the pain, her pain increases. But if you learn to relax properly, letting all muscles become 'limp,' this brings miraculous relief, no matter how intense the contractions. I let myself become so limp I about fell through the bed! With Paulie I had a long first stage—almost fifteen and a half hours, but during this whole time I was so relaxed I didn't feel a bit of pain!"

Carolyn had forgotten all about her mending by now, and a small torn blouse lay untouched in her lap. "Near the end of this stage comes the 'transition' period," she continued. "This is when the baby's head is pushed on through the cervix into the birth canal. These contractions are the longest and the most powerful ones of the whole labor. But by keeping the muscles of the abdomen completely limp as the uterus contracts, you don't have any pain."

Mary leaned forward in her chair. "How can you do that?" she asked breathlessly.

Carolyn smiled. "Well, you see the important thing is to have no muscular resistance to the rise of the uterine contraction. It's important to be lying in the right position, either curled up slightly on the left side, or propped up in the bed in a 'lounge chair' position with pillows under one's knees. A woman should *never* lie on her back in labor! I was comfortable lying on my side, with my knees drawn up and my head bent forward. It was easier to keep my abdomen completely relaxed during contractions this way.

"Then, in this relaxed position, one begins to breathe in and out a little faster than with the 'sleep' breathing. The uterus is working harder and needs more oxygen, so deeper, even, in and out breaths are needed. It is like the 'work' breathing one does when cleaning house or taking a brisk walk, except that only the uterus is working. All the rest of the body must stay limp. At this time the baby's head is pressed against the lower spine, and this can cause a backache. Ralph rubbed my back and it was a big help, but the transition period is *very short*, Mary. It lasts for only six to twelve contractions.

"After these few minutes the baby's head slipped through the cervix into the birth canal, and I felt much better. My backache disappeared. The contractions came farther apart, so I rested limply between them. I felt the urge to bear down with each contraction, and was surprised to find that this not only didn't hurt, but felt good!

"Dr. Gordon had me change then to the 'lounge chair' position. He raised the head of the bed, and had rolled pillows put under my knees. During a contraction he had me take a deep breath in, let it out, take another deep breath and hold it, while I bent forward, curling my back like a letter C. He had me pull my knees back toward my shoulders as I bent over to push down. This is the really exciting time in labor. Dr. Gordon told me to push firmly but not too hard. He reminded me that the vaginal opening has to thin out and open as gently as the cervix did, since forcing it open too fast would make it tear. After about an hour and a half the baby's head began to press against my rectum, and I thought I had to have a bowel movement. I didn't realize that this was my baby! As the head came farther down this sensation completely disappeared, and I began to get a prickly 'pins and needles' sensation as the baby's head bulged against the perineum—that's the outlet you know—and I knew my baby was about to be born. As the outlet stretched further, this prickly sensation disappeared. Dr. Gordon told me this was because the pressure of the baby's head against it had cut off its circulation of blood. Anyway, I couldn't feel anything there. Do you know how it feels when circulation is gradually cut off in your foot—how first it feels tingly, and finally numb? Then you say your foot is 'asleep'?"

Mary nodded, fascinated with what she was learning.

"The outlet is 'asleep' during the actual birth, so all I felt was the bulging pressure of the baby's head which had dilated the birth canal to its fullest capacity. And then I felt the exciting fast passage of his little body moving from the vagina as the birth was completed. The pleasant physical sensations within the birth canal and the emotional climax of this moment were too exciting to describe! Dr. Gordon had me pant in and out as the head was born, so he could control the birth and keep me from tearing, but he let me push the baby's body out—and there was our Paulie!"

Carolyn paused and gazed out the window with a faraway look, recalling that most happy moment which she had experienced three times. Then she finished her story.

"With the baby wrapped in a warmed blanket, and put in my arms at my breast as the afterbirth was delivered (that's the organ in which he lived and was nourished in the womb), I felt I had just taken part in the greatest miracle in the world! I felt like both laughing and crying. I don't like to show my emotions, though, and I think Dr. Gordon has been a little disappointed each time because I am always so quiet. But Ralph! He just acts jubilant! And his excitement spreads to everyone in the room."

"Was there much difference between your first labor and the others?" Mary asked.

"No," Carolyn said, "not in the sensations themselves. With Paulie each stage was much longer but wasn't painful. With Julie and Greg the first stage of labor was so short I barely made it to the hospital, and the second stage lasted only a few minutes." She thought back a moment, smiling to herself.

"I'll have to tell you about the second stage with Paulie. I made such awful grunting noises each time I held my breath to push down—then when I let my breath out slowly after pushing, it would come out in the sound of a moan, rather like a dying cow!"

Mary laughed appreciatively.

"I was really embarrassed to be making so much noise, because I wasn't in any pain at all. I tried to explain this to Ralph, and he squeezed my hand a bit tighter and said, 'I believe you, honey. You've convinced me. Did you know that you're getting red in the face, too, when you push?' I made a face at him for his teasing, but then another contraction came on, and I had to get back to work.

"I was more tired after Paulie's birth, but felt jubilant. After a few hours' rest I felt wonderful. And after Julie's and Greg's births I felt so strong each time that I could have picked up my baby and walked home! Sometimes I've wondered if I wouldn't have been better off just to stay home for the births in the first place."

"I don't know if I'd want my baby to be born at home," Mary mused, "but I want a happy experience like yours. Carolyn, what made you want a natural birth in the first place? I know why *I* want it, because I've always felt in my heart that God made me the way I am, and I'm not afraid to trust Him that He made me the right way. But most people don't understand how I feel."

"There was no one thing, really," Carolyn answered thoughtfully. "I've felt like you, Mary, ever since I was in my teens, but I never had anyone I could talk to about it. Then, one experience of Ralph's and mine really set me to thinking seriously about childbirth. A student from Indonesia spent the day with us, and in the course of our conversation he began to tell us about childbirth customs in his country.

"He said that the Indonesian women would just leave their work in the fields for an hour or so to bear their children, and shortly afterward would be back at work again. But one time he overheard some of their white missionary friends *laughing* among themselves over the way the 'ignorant' Indonesian women gave birth to their babies.

"He seemed very bitter about this. He said he saw no reason why the Indonesian women, who are healthy and muscular from their work in the fields, should go home to bear their children and suffer like the missionary women. He told us that the Indonesian women he knew accept childbirth as a perfectly normal process, and it doesn't seem to trouble them.

"That conversation set me to thinking," Carolyn said. "What about the 'curse of Eve' tradition? If God meant for *all* women to suffer in giving birth, why did the Indonesian women escape it but not the missionary women? Then, one day when I was doing visitation for our church, I stopped at the house of a Chinese family."

Mary sat listening in rapt attention.

"Several of the children in this family were in our Sunday school. The mother looked so young I could hardly believe that she had *ten* children! Her last baby was only a week old, and while the other little ones tumbled about on the floor, one child who had been in my class climbed into my lap and put her arms around me as the mother told me all about her latest birth experience.

" 'Usually it's nothing,' she told me, 'you know, just a *push, push* —like a *one, two.*' She said she could deliver her babies by herself and had always gone about her daily work the day after a child was born. But she had always called in a midwife—just in case something should go wrong.

"Two of her babies were born before the midwife arrived, and she had delivered them and taken care of them by herself. She was *most* annoyed that she'd still had to pay the midwife the regular fee just the same!

"But this time, she said, she was glad the midwife came as the baby was 'a-reverse.' At first I didn't understand what she meant, but she gestured with her hands as if she were holding something and turning it over. Then I realized she meant that she'd had a breech baby—its little bottom presented first, instead of its head.

"She told how her husband had been assisting at the birth. Once the midwife asked him to put the lubricating cream on her sterile gloves, but he squirted so much from the tube that her hands kept slipping as she tried to turn the baby's position to make the birth easier. This little Chinese mother beamed as she told how they had all laughed over this and how the midwife had had to change her gloves so that she could try again.

"I could hardly believe my ears! Here she had been in the midst of a most difficult delivery, and yet she said that she had been *laughing!* So I asked her if she had ever had any anesthesia.

"She was completely puzzled by the word at first. Then she understood and shook her head. Mary, I can't tell you how I felt that day! Here she'd had a breech baby, and had to work so hard that she said she'd been too 'tired' to take over her full household responsibilities until the baby was three days old!

"Her cheerful, normal attitude toward giving birth made a profound impression on me. I couldn't help thinking of Sarah in the Bible—bearing a child when she was an old, old woman, who yet said, 'God hath made me to *laugh*, so that all that hear will laugh with me.'

"My interest was really aroused now," Carolyn continued. "It was right after my visit with the Chinese lady that I turned completely away from any confidence in 'orthodox' obstetrics, and began to study the natural childbirth philosophy in earnest. I began to look for more items about how native women bear their children. I read, for example, that the Laotian women bear their babies more easily than we do, although some of their customs don't add to the mother's comfort—like having their husbands blow in their ears throughout their labor, so the baby will have enough air!"

Just then Julie appeared in the doorway, pink-cheeked and warm from her nap. Seeing Mary, she came to her shyly, and let Mary lift her onto her lap. Carolyn excused herself a moment to check the baby, but he was still asleep. As she came back into the room she was turning the pages of a book.

"I began thumbing through books on anthropology," she said, "to try to find some explanation for women suffering in our culture, but not in many of the others. Margaret Mead, the well-known anthropologist, says the majority of women suffer severe pain in childbirth, *or* accept giving birth matter-of-factly, depending on the culture in which they live. She says that pain, when it occurs, is not due to the physiology of the birth process, but to the attitudes toward birth which a woman has 'learned' from her culture. Listen to this!" Carolyn sat down and began to read from the page she had marked:

So child-birth may be experienced according to the phrasing given it by the culture, as an experience that is dangerous and painful, interesting and engrossing, matter-of-fact and mildly hazardous. . . . Whether they are allowed to see births or not, men contribute their share to the way in which child-birth is viewed, and I have seen male informants writhe on the floor, in magnificent pantomime of a painful delivery, who have never themselves seen or heard a woman in labour. . . . Men who feel copulation as aggressive may have different phantasies about the dire effects on their wives of their dreadful uncontrolled aggressive desires from men who feel copulation as pleasant, who may share in a cultural phrasing which insists that the child "sleeps quietly until it is time to be born, then puts its hands above its head and comes out." . . .

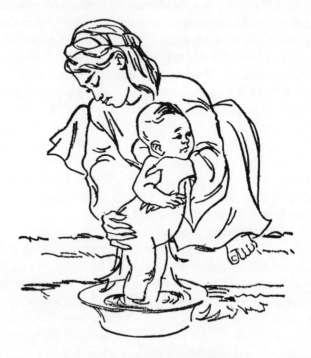

Fig. 1. Vietnamese mother squatting to give her baby a roadside bath. Notice how she sits right on her heels, her knees wide apart. This drawing is a copy of a photograph.

It cannot be argued that child-birth is both an unbearable pain and a bearable pain, both a situation from which all women naturally shrink in dread and a situation towards which all women naturally move readily and happily, both a danger to be avoided and a consummation devoutly to be desired. At least one aspect must be regarded as learned. . . . There seems some reason to believe that the male imagination, undisciplined and uninformed by immediate bodily clues or immediate bodily experiences, may have contributed disproportionately to the cultural super-structure of belief and practice regarding childbearing. It is perhaps not without significance that in those Polynesian societies where the male participates in his wife's delivery as a husband, not as a magician or a priest, there is an extremely simple, uncomplicated attitude towards birth; women do not scream, but instead *work,* and men need no self-imposed expiatory activities afterwards.[1]

"Why, then," Mary exclaimed, understanding the point, "for a woman to experience severe pain in childbirth depends on whether or not she has been conditioned by the culture she lives in to expect it!" She thought a moment, frowning. "But what about the teaching of the Bible? Doesn't it say that God has condemned *all* the women of the world to suffer in childbirth because of Eve?"

"This'll surprise you, Mary," Carolyn said emphatically, "but the Bible doesn't say that at all! This was a problem to me, too, so I took it to Pastor Dirkson. He looked up the meaning of all the Hebrew and Greek words used about childbirth in the Bible, and he discovered that there is *nothing* there which says women are meant to suffer pain when they bear a child. I want you and John to go ask him about this. He can explain it much better than I can.

"Incidentally, Mary, it's interesting that it's we mothers who can really promote natural childbirth. Doctors have seen so many women suffer that they hesitate to believe a birth is possible without it. And preachers—well, how can they go around telling women they shouldn't be suffering in childbirth when they are? But we women can, because we *know!*"

"Carolyn," Mary said, as she put Julie down and rose to leave, "I just can't tell you how much this day has meant to me! I thought I was the only woman in the world who felt the way I do about having babies—but now I know I have lots of company!"

Notes

1. Margaret Mead, *Male and Female* (New York: Morrow, 1949), pp. 236–38. Reprinted by permission.

Chapter 7

A Kindness in His Justice

*Oh that men would praise the Lord for his
goodness, and for his wonderful works to
the children of men!* Ps. 107:8.

Mary and John were not aware of the threadbare carpet on the
living room floor of the parsonage, worn thin by the feet of many
seekers after counsel and hope. Nor did they notice the many
patiently mended little places in the faded curtains hanging over
the old-fashioned bay window. But they were aware of the crackling fire in the fireplace shedding a warmth throughout the room
and of something undefinable in the peaceful atmosphere of this
home that made them feel at ease.

"This is delicious nut bread, Mrs. Dirkson," Mary remarked.

"Thank you, Mary," replied the pastor's wife. "Would you care
for more coffee?"

"No, thanks. I'm still not a very good cook, although John is
quite patient with me."

"She's being modest," John defended her. "I haven't complained,
have I, Mary? The only thing I've really missed is lemon pie like
Aunt Em makes."

"I don't know much about pies," Mary admitted, "so I've been
afraid to try—but some day I'll surprise you!"

"I'll be glad to show you how, Mary," Mrs. Dirkson offered, "if
you'll come over some morning. It's not so hard once you've

learned how." Just then Pastor Dirkson came in the back door. "Come on in the living room, Carl," his wife called. "John and Mary are already here."

The pastor hung up his coat and came into the room. "Sorry I've kept you waiting," he said, nodding a greeting to them both. He took a chair near the fire, leaning forward to warm his hands. "I paid Mrs. Arkwright a call this evening, but it's hard to break away from her, so I'm later than I'd intended to be. Poor soul— she's so lonely."

"Mother goes over to see her quite often," Mary said. "I suppose I could stop by once in a while, too."

"She'd certainly appreciate a visit. That's enough coffee, Ruth." He finished the slice of nut bread his wife had served him and reached for his Bible. "I understand you've come to see me about the same problem that worried Carolyn Thebes. Is that right?"

"Yes," John replied. "Mary told me about her visit with Carolyn the other day, and this question about the Bible saying that God cursed all women with pain in childbirth really came out into the open. Carolyn said she'd gone over this problem with you and wanted us to come talk to you.

"We had quite a discussion with Mary's folks one day," John went on, "about the three basic causes for suffering. We felt that these three were, first, the sinful acts of people which as often as not cause suffering to the innocent; second, calamities of nature; and, third, the presence of an evil force at work in our world. But we don't know where the 'curse of Eve' would fit into this summary."

"That's a good summary, John," the pastor told him. "I assume that by the 'curse of Eve,' you mean that women have been given an unfair punishment of physical pain, while man has been allowed to get by with the lighter punishment of tilling the ground?"

John nodded, so Pastor Dirkson told him, "God didn't discriminate unfairly against women at the outset of our Bible! I've studied every passage in the Bible pertaining to childbirth and checked the English translations against the original languages, and I've found that *there is not one single verse in the entire Bible which mentions any 'curse' on Eve, or on all womankind.* On the contrary, a 'curse' is only mentioned as being on those women who did *not* bear a child. In the Bible, the mother of children is portrayed as a woman blessed by God; the barren woman as a woman whom God had judged. Even centuries later, after the time of Christ, this concept was still true among Jews and Christians alike. In an apocryphal account of Anna, the mother of Mary, there's an example of this. Anna's maid berates her in this way:

> "I cannot wish you a greater curse than you are under, in that God hath shut up your womb, that you should not be a mother in Israel."[1]

The pastor was warming to his subject now, guilty at times of "sermonizing" in his conversation.

"The common interpretation of the 'curse of Eve' is based on one lone verse in the Bible, found in the third chapter of Genesis where the sin of Adam and Eve is recorded. But think back to Eden a moment. After Adam and Eve had sinned, did a wrathful God come storming into the garden in a rage to wreak vengeance on their heads?

"Not at all! A compassionate Creator came calling them, searching for the sinners. It was *man* who had broken fellowship with God, who was no longer at ease in God's holy presence, and who had hidden himself!

"The revelation of God's great love for sinners begins in Eden. The message of Calvary begins in Eden. God's longing for the sinner to be restored to fellowship with Himself, ultimately led to His great sacrifice of His own Son, to pay the penalty for man's sin. And as a loving God came calling, seeking to re-establish communion with the sinners in the garden, so He's still calling all mankind, longing to restore to fellowship with Himself all who'll accept His forgiveness through Calvary. This is the central message of the Bible, the very core of Christianity:

> For God so loved the world, that he gave his only begotten Son, that whosoever believeth in him should not perish, but have everlasting life.

For as in Adam all die, even so in Christ shall all be made alive.

"But God, though He loved Adam and Eve, and through them the whole human race, and though He provided a means for their forgiveness, still found it necessary to impose a discipline upon them in this temporal life. Turn with me now, please, to Genesis 3:16 and 17."

John opened his own Bible to this passage, sharing it with Mary as the pastor began reading from the Authorized Version, pointing out the underlying Hebrew word which was of significance:

> Unto the woman he said, I will greatly multiply thy *sorrow* (**etsev**) and thy conception; in *sorrow* (**etsev**) thou shalt bring forth children.

"Do you notice that the word 'curse' is not used here, and neither is the word 'pain'? But now, let's compare what God said to Eve with what He says to Adam in the following verse:

> And unto Adam he said, . . . cursed is the ground for thy sake; in *sorrow* (**etsev**) shalt thou eat of it all the days of thy life."

"The Hebrew words are the *same* for the man and the woman!" Mary exclaimed.

"Yes, they are. But have you never noticed that the English words, 'sorrow' for Eve, and 'sorrow' for Adam are also the same? Notice, too, in the context, that the word 'cursed' is used of the *ground*, and of the *serpent*, but not of Adam or Eve. Look now, in the margin[2] of your Bible, at the alternate translation for 'sorrow' in reference to Adam. What is it?"

"It says 'toil,' " Mary answered, looking over John's arm to read the smaller print. "That means hard work. Why, pastor!" she exclaimed again, "that's exactly what Carolyn told me giving birth is like. She said it's hard work! But why is the word 'toil' not in the margin for the woman too, since the Hebrew word is the same for her as for Adam?"

"There's no good reason, Mary," he told her, "except that our translators are influenced by our own culture. You see, a translator sometimes unconsciously gives words a very different meaning from that intended by the original author, simply because he lives in a different era, a different culture, and has from childhood looked at many phases of life from a different philosophical point of view. This is one reason we must never discontinue the study of the Bible in the original languages."

"Carolyn and I talked about the attitude toward childbirth being different in different cultures," Mary said, seeing his point.

"Yes, that's very true. In the last hundred years especially, Biblical scholars have become more and more aware of the need for recognizing cultural differences in the lives of the people of Bible times from aspects of our Western culture. But, unfortunately, they haven't had enough knowledge of anthropology to realize that there are cultural differences in attitudes toward childbearing also. Thus Bible translators and scholars have mistakenly assumed that childbirth is the same the world over and that every mention of it in the Bible meant to the Hebrew women exactly what it means to their own wives in their present culture.

"But what about the culture of Moses' day and the experiences of the women of that time? We should remember that the Hebrews were what we would call a more primitive race. They were an agricultural, nomadic people, and the sense of 'family' was very strong. Large families are considered a blessing in most agricultural societies, and the Hebrews considered a woman who had given birth to many children to be highly honored."

"Carolyn also explained to me that many primitive women give birth more easily and matter-of-factly than in our culture," Mary interrupted him.

"That's another good point. Samuel Zwemer, an early missionary to the Arabs, says that Arab women didn't have painful deliveries until *after* their society had been adversely affected by Western culture. Even when trekking across the desert, an Arab woman simply dropped behind the caravan when her labor began. After giving birth to her infant in the sand she would walk, some-

times for many hours, to overtake the caravan, carrying her baby.
The experiences of the Hebrew women of the Pentateuch were
surely similar to these, since they were of the same Semitic origin
and culture.

"Now let's come back to this Hebrew word *etsev* in Genesis,
keeping the Hebrew culture in mind. A Hebrew rabbi, Samson
Hirsch, who lived a hundred years ago, has carefully explained the
meaning of this word. He says that *etsev* refers *only* to a mental
state, specifically, to that of 'renunciation,' or a 'giving up' of
oneself, as in toil.[3]

"Rabbi Hirsch was careful to point out to the Jewish people of
his generation that God had used the same word, *etsev*, for Eve,
as for Adam! He says too, that God disciplined them not *because*
they had sinned but '*for their sakes*.' Eve was to toil to bring forth
the fruit of the body, Adam was to toil to bring forth the fruit of
the ground, that they might learn to appreciate the good gifts that
had been so freely given them before."

"It's still true, isn't it," John observed, "that we don't really
appreciate the things we get for nothing, without lifting a finger?"

"Yes, it is, John. This discipline of working for what we receive
is really a blessing in disguise.

"Now Rabbi Hirsch also points out most emphatically that the
Jews have *never* believed that there was any 'curse' on Adam and
Eve but only on the ground and on the serpent. The earliest Chris-
tians also make this same distinction.

"But there is something else I'd like you to notice, before we
turn to one passage in the New Testament. Ruth, would you please
hand me my copy of the Revised Standard Version?" His wife
handed it to him.

"This is a very recent translation of the Bible," he explained.
"Listen:

> To the woman he said, 'I will greatly multiply your *pain* (**etsev**)
> in childbearing; in *pain* (**etsev**) you shall bring forth chil-
> dren, . . .
> And to Adam he said, . . . "cursed is the ground because of
> you; in *toil* (**etsev**) shall you eat of it all the days of your life."

"What right did they have to do that!" John exclaimed indignantly, "—translating *pain* for the woman and *toil* for the man, when the Hebrew word is the same for them both!"

Pastor Dirkson smiled. "Remember what I said to you about translators 'reading into' a word from another language their own understanding of it, because of cultural differences? That's exactly what's been done here. The common belief, in our culture, is that the birth of a child always causes its mother great pain.

"Now, there's a verse in the New Testament about childbirth that I'd like you to look at a moment—or shall we wait and take this up another time?"

"Oh, no," Mary said eagerly, "please, let's go on."

"All right. This is a statement made by Our Lord in John 16:21 and 22." He waited until John had found the passage in his Bible before reading:

> A woman when she is in travail hath sorrow, because her hour is come: but as soon as she is delivered of the child, she remembereth no more the anguish, for joy that a man has been born into the world.
>
> And ye now therefore have sorrow: but I will see you again, and your hearts will rejoice, and your joy no man taketh from you.

"I don't understand these verses!" Mary admitted.

"Neither do I, Mary," John told her, "at least not until the pastor explains them."

"This verse is poorly translated," Pastor Dirkson said, "as you will realize in a moment. The words translated 'in travail' are from the Greek word *tiktō*, which simply means, 'to bring forth a child.' For example, this same word is used in Luke of the birth of Christ:

> And she *brought forth* (**tiktō**) her first born son, and wrapped him in swaddling clothes. . . .

"The word 'sorrow' is from the Greek word *lupē*, which, like *etsev*, refers only to a state of the emotions.[4] Historical records just prior to Christ's time reveal that a birth during this period in history generally took only two to three hours, so we can be certain that Christ is not speaking of the 'sorrow' of a prolonged, painful, delivery."

"Could He be referring to the sorrow of exertion in giving birth?" Mary asked.

"It seems possible, Mary," the pastor nodded. "After all, giving birth is a task requiring complete, sober absorption. *Lupē* might also refer here to the mother's anxiety in her labor, until the task had been successfully accomplished.

"In this passage Jesus is using a parallel similar to that in Genesis between man and woman, only here, He compares a woman's experience of giving birth to the disciples' coming experience of waiting in sorrow for His release from the grave. But the comparison is not primarily of the sorrow, but of the *joy* which is to follow.

"It's most revealing that Christ is aware of the tremendous *joy*, or *elation*, which a mother experiences immediately after a normal birth. This is not just a state of being 'happy' that 'it's all over' and the child has arrived safely, but it is an exhilaration which sweeps from her mind all thought of whatever anxiety or weariness of toil she may have experienced—'she remembereth it no more!' This exciting climax to the birth experience is a most important part of it, and gives it the needed balance. We see in this, as in so many other things, the wise and loving plan of our great Creator. In Christ's day, because the women didn't experience real suffering in a normal birth, nor were their minds dulled by drugs at this final moment of birth, they *did* experience this sense of exaltation immediately afterward, as He tells us.

"But there's one more word in this verse that's mistranslated. It's the word 'anguish' from the Greek word *thlipsis*, which means simply, 'applying pressure, compressing together, or squeezing,' as in squeezing out the grapes, or in pushing someone out of his place."[5]

"Then you mean that Jesus said the mother no longer remembers pushing the baby out of his place!" exclaimed Mary excitedly.

"Yes, Mary. That's exactly what Jesus said. In Latin translations of this verse *thlipsis* is translated as *pressurae,* meaning, the 'pres-

sures' of childbirth. This is a common word to use of childbirth
for these people, as for example in the apocryphal account of the
birth of Christ where Mary says to Joseph:

> Take me down from off the ass, for that which is in me *presses*
> to come forth. . . . Then said Mary again to Joseph, Take me
> down, for that which is within me *mightily presses* me.[6]

"Do you see how she felt her baby being pressed, pushed down,
by the uterus? Now, let's translate John 16:21 literally and see
what impression it makes:

> A woman when she is *giving birth* (**tiktō**) has *sorrow* (**lupē**)
> because her hour is come: but as soon as she has given birth
> to the child, she no longer remembers the *pressures* (**thlipsis**)
> for joy that a child has been born into the world."

"That's a beautiful verse!" Mrs. Dirkson commented. She had
listened quietly all evening, only slipping out of her place unobtrusively from time to time to stir up the embers of the fire, to
keep it burning brightly.

"It is indeed beautiful," her husband agreed. "But what do you
think the real emphasis of this whole passage might be?"

All were silent a moment, thinking, until John suggested, "Isn't
Jesus trying to comfort His disciples? He knows He's going to die,
and He's trying to get them to look beyond the sorrow they'll
experience at His death, to the great joy they'll know when His
resurrection takes place."

"Good, John," pastor said, pleased. "Jesus draws from an
example they all know—the excited joy of a new mother just after
the birth of her child—to *comfort* their hearts. He pictures the
mother giving birth, no doubt groaning in her bearing down efforts
to push her child out of his place within her body. Suddenly her
task is completed, as her child breaks forth from the dark womb
into life. With a glad cry, and unbelieving tears of laughter, she
takes into her arms the wonderful reward of her labor—her very
own live, perfect baby!

"Jesus is drawing from the moment of a most intense joy in human experience, to illustrate the intense joy His disciples will know, when He Himself breaks forth from the dark tomb into new life—in the power and glory of the Resurrection!"

"I've gained a new respect for the Bible tonight," John remarked thoughtfully. "We surely thank you for the time you've taken to explain these things, pastor. I suppose there's more you could tell us about this?"

"Oh, yes, a great deal more," he smiled, "but we'll save that for another time." He walked with John and Mary to the door, after they had slipped into their wraps, and held it open for them.

"Good night, Mrs. Dirkson," Mary called back, "and thank you for the refreshments."

"You're most welcome, both of you. Good night."

Long after John had gone to sleep that night, Mary lay awake in the dark thinking over what she had learned that evening. She felt fully released from the anxiety in her mind that God had condemned her to pain—an anxious burden that women like herself had carried for centuries. The words and melody of a lovely hymn came to her mind, and as it echoed over and over, she gradually drifted away into the most peaceful slumber that she had ever known.

> There's a wideness in God's mercy,
>   Like the wideness of the sea;
> There's a kindness in His justice,
>   Which is more than liberty.
>
> For the love of God is broader
>   Than the measure of man's mind;
> And the heart of the Eternal
>   Is most wonderfully kind.
>
> If our love were but more simple
>   We would take Him at His word,
> And our lives would be all sunshine
>   In the sweetness of our Lord.[7]

Notes

1. *Protevangelion of James* 2:6, 7.
2. The Oxford Self-Pronouncing Bible, Teacher's Edition, Authorized Version.
3. Rabbi Samson Raphael Hirsch, *The Pentateuch* (a translation and commentary), Vol. I, Genesis, rendered into English by the publisher (London: Isaac Levy, 1959).
4. Arndt, W. F. and Gingrich, F. W., eds. *A Greek-English Lexicon of the New Testament, and Other Early Christian Literature* (Chicago: University of Chicago Press, 1957).
5. *Ibid.*
6. *Protevangelion of James* 12:10–12.
7. Frederick Faber, "There's a Wideness in God's Mercy."

Chapter 8

Smaller than a Hand

He shall feed his flock like a shepherd: he shall gather the lambs with his arm, and carry them in his bosom, and shall gently lead those that are with young. Isa. 40:11.

The clapboards of the tiny frame house clung tenaciously together. The overgrown weeds in the scraggly yard lent an air of desertion, but a curtain shifted at the window as Mary and her mother came up the walk. It was evident that someone lived in this forlorn little brown house.

"I must get Dad over here some Saturday to nail up those loose boards," Mrs. Johnson remarked to her daughter.

"John can come trim the yard when Dad comes," Mary said, generously offering her husband's services, too, without his knowing it. "It's a good thing it rains so much here, isn't it, Mother? At least it keeps the yard green."

As Mary lifted her hand, she was startled by the door opening suddenly, before she'd had time to touch the doorbell.

"I saw you folks a-comin' up the walk," Mrs. Arkwright told them. "I sit by the window and watch, most days, for someone to come see me. I get so lonely now with Mr. Arkwright gone!" She brushed an invisible tear from her cheek with her gnarled hand as she led them into the little house, which smelled faintly of stale grease and fried onions.

Mary wrinkled her nose at the musty odors as she and her mother sat down. It's funny, she thought to herself, as she looked around the room—that I don't remember this place as being so dirty. All I can remember is that Jo Lynn and I always were given a piece of candy from that blue bowl when we came with Mother to visit. I suppose there were dust balls under the furniture and that the window sills were gray with dirt then, too, and we just didn't notice it.

"It's a lovely day today, isn't it?" Mary's mother said pleasantly to Mrs. Arkwright, after they had been seated.

"I'm very well, thank you," the old lady replied, misunderstanding, "except I git a bit more pain in my shoulders with this cold weather. My, Mary! how you've grown!" She looked Mary up and down unabashedly. "You're quite the young lady now, ain't you though!"

"I'm *married* now," said Mary, not too politely, annoyed at being spoken to like a child.

"Eh?"

"I'm married now," Mary answered, speaking louder.

"Eh? Eh? What's that?" Mrs. Arkwright looked questioningly at Mary's mother.

"SHE'S MARRIED NOW," Mrs. Johnson shouted, and Mrs. Arkwright nodded happily.

"Married! Well, I declare! Seems just the other day you and Jo Lynn was a-skippin' up the walk to see me. Married! D'you have any kiddies yet?"

"We're going to have a baby next spring," Mary replied loudly.

"How nice! A baby! Well, I declare! Is it a boy or a girl?"

"No—ah, we don't know," said Mary lamely, then, gathering her courage she said, more loudly still, "It hasn't been BORN yet."

"A boy!" exclaimed Mrs. Arkwright with delight. "Now ain't that nice!" She stopped rocking as Mrs. Johnson leaned over and shouted in her ear.

"THE BABY HASN'T BEEN BORN YET."

"Oh, not born yet. Well, I declare. Excuse me a minute," she said, fumbling with her hearing aid, "I don't believe this thing's workin' just right. I can't seem to hear you." She eased herself out of the rocker and limped into the next room, calling back over her shoulder, "I'll see if I can find a better battery."

"You'd think she'd know, Mother," Mary whispered, "I *am* wearing a maternity dress."

"You're still quite slender though, Mary," her mother soothed her ruffled feelings. "Mrs. Arkwright lost track of styles long ago. She doesn't know a maternity dress from any other unless a girl is very obviously pregnant."

They could hear an eerie collection of squeaks, whistles, and static coming from the next room, as Mrs. Arkwright shuffled through a drawer full of hearing-aid batteries and tested them.

"She's trying to find a good battery," Mary's mother explained. "She never knows the new ones from the old, so she has to test them all."

"But doesn't the county keep her supplied with good ones?" Mary asked.

"Yes, but you see, she never throws the old ones away, as she's so afraid she'll run out of them altogether some day. But this way she gets them all mixed up. She'll probably come back with an older one than she had before."

After what seemed an interminable length of time, Mrs. Arkwright reappeared, apparently satisfied with the battery she had chosen. She was carrying a yellowed bit of cloth in her hands. "I've got something for your baby," she told Mary. "I love babies! This little dress was left from our Betsy who died of the dipytheria." She smoothed out the little dress with her stiffened, arthritic fingers, as she placed it in Mary's lap. "There's nobody I'd ruther give it to than you, Mary. Your mother's always been so good to me."

Mary nodded a gracious thank you to her, having been notified by a look in her mother's eye that she dare not refuse the gift. As she opened the musty folds, she saw that it had been lovely once, painstakingly embroidered, with tatted lace around the sleeves and hem. She folded it again, and laid it gently in her lap.

"Would you care to have some tea?" Mrs. Arkwright offered.

"No, thank you," Mary answered, but her mother was already saying,

"YES, WE WOULD ENJOY IT."

Mrs. Arkwright hobbled out into the little kitchen to put the water on to boil, obviously pleased that they would stay.

"Mother, why did you say that!" Mary scolded. "You know we can't stay much longer. I have to be home when John gets there, so we'll be on time for the doctor's appointment."

"This won't take long, Mary. Did you see how happy she was when we said we'd love to have tea with her? You see, it gives such pleasure to people like her to be able to do some little thing for others, because they have so few chances to repay the many favors done for them."

After another lengthy delay, Mrs. Arkwright returned with a tray. She set it down on the table near Mrs. Johnson. Although she filled the cups as carefully as she could, her hands trembled so much that a little tea splashed out of each one.

"It's kind of you folks to bring me the berry pie. I thought you might's well share it, as I don't eat so very much. These here are wildberries, ain't they?"

Mrs. Johnson nodded in the affirmative.

"Thank you for the tea, Mrs. Arkwright," Mary shouted, when they had finished their repast. "We really must be getting home in a little while."

"Go home with you a little while?" Mrs. Arkwright cried, her face creasing into a thousand tiny wrinkles as she beamed at Mary. "Why, if you ain't the sweetest thing! I'd be delighted! Just a minute. I'll go get my wraps."

"Mother!" Mary cried in dismay, as Mrs. Arkwright fumbled in the closet for her coat, "what'll I do now!"

Mrs. Johnson couldn't help smiling. "Don't worry, dear. Leave her off at my house instead while you and John go to the doctor. You can take her home again on your way back. It'll do her good to get out."

"Are you too warm, Mary?" John questioned her in concern. She was lying on the examining table waiting for the doctor to come in, and John had noticed that her cheeks were very flushed.

"I'm all right," she said, "I'm just a little unnerved from the visit with Mrs. Arkwright. She's such a *character,* John!" The doctor entered the examining room while she was speaking.

"Did I hear Mrs. Arkwright's name?" he asked as he greeted them. He, too, noticed Mary's flushed look. "She's a 'character,' all right, Mary. She'd feel much better if she'd take the medicines I prescribe for her, but she prefers her own home remedies most of the time. Diagnoses her own troubles, too—like three-fourths of my women patients, I might add." John laughed appreciatively, and Mary relaxed her tensions a bit.

"You're looking well, Mary," he observed, as he touched her hand gently for a moment. As he had expected, it was cold, and her palms were moist with perspiration. Her tension was obvious to him.

"I've never felt better," she replied, "but I still haven't felt the baby move. It's about time for that, isn't it?"

"Soon now, I should think. Usually the baby quickens around the eighteenth week of pregnancy. I should be able to hear his heartbeat today, though." He placed his stethoscope over her abdomen and listened intently, moving it two or three times. "It's there, all right. Want to listen, John?"

John awkwardly placed the stethoscope on the spot the doctor indicated. He listened carefully, and moved the instrument gingerly a time or two without success.

"You'll be able to hear it next month," Dr. Gordon reassured him, "when the heartbeat's stronger. We'll let Mary listen then, too."

"How big is the baby now?" John asked, handing the stethoscope back to the doctor.

"Hold out your hand," was the reply. As John did so, the doctor said, "The baby would fit into the curve of your hand. At four months, it's between six and seven inches long, and weighs about four and a quarter ounces."

"Smaller than a hand," John said wonderingly, looking at his own. In imagination he could feel the weight of the little body snuggled into his palm.

"Now Mary," the doctor said, turning back to her, "let's see how well you've learned to relax. Take a deep relaxed breath, please, and let it out slowly."

Try as she would, Mary could not, and began blushing still more. The harder she tried to breathe slowly and deeply in the diaphragm, the more rapidly she breathed in and out with her upper chest.

"I honestly have been practicing, doctor," she said, dismayed.

"Can you relax your hand?" he asked, lifting it by the wrist. Her hand swung stiffly back and forth as he shook it gently. "Let it hang loosely," he told her, and she relaxed it a bit more. "It's still too tense. Let it go *completely limp,* so I can shake it like an old dishrag." Mary obeyed, and as her hand relaxed, she unconsciously took her first slow deep breath also.

"Good!" he encouraged her. "Now we're getting somewhere." Mary began breathing more deeply and more rhythmically, relaxing her tensions more and more.

"You have the right idea, Mary," Dr. Gordon encouraged her, "but you must learn to release your tensions much more quickly. Sit up a moment now, and I'll explain what I mean." He took her hand, and helped her to a sitting position.

"I purposely tested Mary's ability to relax first today," he explained to them both, "to illustrate what tension is, so you can recognize it. I realized as soon as I came into the room, by the unusual color in her cheeks, by her cold, moist hands, and by her rapid breathing—we call it 'hyperventilating'—that Mary was in a mild state of anxiety, although outwardly she acted very calm. If you were to go into labor with just this much tension, Mary, and be unable to release it, you'd soon be in pain, because tension inhibits the normal progress of the birth.

"Here's an exaggerated example of what tension does. Suppose you're crossing the street with a small child, who suddenly darts away from you, just as an ambulance comes screeching around the corner, sirens going full blast. In that instant, the blood rushes to your head, your heart beats faster, you breathe rapidly, and many of your normal body processes, such as digestion, are temporarily inhibited. A mild state of tension produces all these same symptoms, only in a modified form.

"But why are you tense today, Mary? You've known me all your life. You're not afraid of me?"

"No," she said.

"But you're a little anxious about the examination today?"

Mary nodded.

"You're not alone in this," he smiled reassuringly. "Most young women, coming in for a first internal examination, feel just as you do. They aren't sure just what the doctor will do, they're embarrassed at the thought of a vaginal examination, and they tense to cover their anxiety with an appearance of poise. Is this how you feel?"

"Well, yes," Mary admitted, "I can't help being a little nervous about it."

"I'm glad you're honest with me, Mary. Let your bit of anxiety today be an object lesson for you, of *the same state of tension* in which nearly all women about to have their first babies enter the unfamiliar surroundings of a modern hospital. Remember what I said to you about the natural shyness of a young woman, John?"

John nodded, understanding.

"Tension due to the simple embarrassment of a young wife in labor can be a tremendous pain-producing factor. The primitive woman giving birth out in the fields, or in her own little hut, suffers no such embarrassment. And a young woman can overcome her reticence, and gain the poise and self-confidence she needs for this experience if she's prepared beforehand. Now, Mary," he added, "I'll explain what I'm going to do today, so you needn't feel anxious or embarrassed.

"We'll do a routine physical first, such as I've often done for you. Then we'll measure the bones of your pelvis to see if they're of adequate size to permit a normal delivery. Then I'll examine you internally by means of an instrument like this." He picked up a small cylindrical instrument and handed it to her.

"This is called a speculum," he said, as she turned it over in her hands, "and it's used to hold the vaginal walls apart so that I can examine the cervix inside your body. I do very much the same thing when I use a tongue depressor to hold down your tongue when I look at your throat. The cervix, you know, is the little doorway into the uterus, so it's important for me to know that it's in good condition. If you take deep abdominal breaths, as you've been doing, and keep the vaginal walls relaxed, the speculum won't cause you any discomfort."

Mary looked relieved. "Well, is that all there is to it! I'm glad you told me. Will you examine the cervix each time I come in from now on?"

"No, just this first time, and possibly on a few occasions near the end of your pregnancy."

"There's one other thing that really worries me, doctor," Mary said, as she handed the speculum to John to look over. "How do I know that my baby will be all right? I've heard so many things about stillborn babies and babies born with mind defects."

Fig. 2. The speculum.

"That'll take time to answer," he replied, as he proceeded with the examination, "so let's wait and discuss it in my office a bit later."

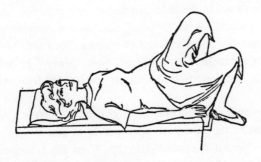

Fig. 3. Patient in position for a pelvic examination.

"Now to come back to your question, Mary . . ." Dr. Gordon said, as he slipped into his chair behind the desk. John and Mary had been waiting in his office for several minutes, while he had been busy with other patients. The doctor looked weary as he ran his fingers through his graying hair, wondering how he should go about telling these young people what they wanted to know.

"I have some more instructions for you today, Mary," he said first, as he handed her another small folder. "Please study them carefully and do as they say."

"I certainly will," she said earnestly.

"Now, you should both realize," he began, "that there is always a possibility of abnormality in a new baby. At the same time, I would reassure you that you are both doing a great deal toward making it possible for your baby to be normal and healthy by preparing for him to be born naturally.

"Do you know that there are thirteen other countries in the world which have a *lower* death rate for babies than the United States? In all these other nations, natural childbirth is more widely practiced than in our country. In the United States, for example, we lose almost twice as many babies per thousand live births as in Sweden. It has been estimated that 60 per cent of the infant deaths in the United States are attributable to lack of sufficient oxygen during birth, partly because of improper use of drugs."

"Why, doctor!" exclaimed Mary. "I thought the United States was way ahead of all other countries in the fields of medicine!"

"This is true of many of our medical specialties," he said, "but it's a proven fact that in obstetrics our nation is about twenty years behind. I was shocked when I read a statement in a national magazine not long ago that infant deaths due to childbirth are the fifth major cause of mortality in this country.[1] The same article went on to say that sixty thousand babies a year are damaged during birth— only to survive with cerebral palsy, epilepsy, or some degree of mental crippling. Our country has a greater percentage of cerebral-palsied children in proportion to our population than any other nation in the world! It makes one wonder what cultural and environmental factors in the United States would cause such a deplorable record. Several years ago *Medical Times* published an article on birth injuries by the late Dr. J. Lawrence Cochran, in which he mentioned the statement of a neurosurgeon that 70 per cent of these American children were crippled at birth."[2]

"That's a disgrace!" John exploded.

"Indeed it is," Dr. Gordon agreed. "Another very sad thing is that mothers in our country die so needlessly in childbirth. Anesthetic deaths have been ranked as one of the leading causes of maternal mortality. In a single study of over eight thousand maternal deaths, two-thirds of them were listed as preventable.

"Another thing that saddens me is the depression of so many new mothers who've been drugged, following the birth of their children. Some doctors claim that this is a 'natural' result of the effort and excitement of giving birth, but we don't feel depressed after the excitement of strenuous exercise, do we?"

"Certainly not!" John agreed. "You feel physically tired but emotionally refreshed."

"There's no proven physiological reason for the depression of so many new mothers in the United States.[3] Their depression often springs from an inner resentment, which they can't identify.[4] A mother may even secretly reject her child, although she guiltily struggles to conceal this fact, even from herself.

"One other tragic fact is that far too many of our American babies unnecessarily become mentally defective,[5] as I mentioned. Research is gaining momentum in this area, and the facts that are being discovered are sobering indeed. And how many of our children are there who are not actually mentally defective, but whose intelligence is below normal, who are poor readers, but who might have been as bright and normal as their brothers and sisters[6] if they had not received some slight damage to their higher brain cells because of the drugs and anesthetics used as they were being born, or medications unnecessarily given during pregnancy?"[7]

"Doctor," Mary said, as seriously as she had ever spoken in her life, "I'll do anything you say in order to give birth to my baby without the use of these things!"

"I know you will, Mary, and I'll do all I know to help you. Remember, though, that there *is* a place for the proper use of analgesics and anesthetics in childbirth. In an emergency they may be lifesaving to mother and child alike, and if this occurred I would be compelled to administer an anesthetic, whether you wanted it or not. Even Dr. Dick-Read found it necessary to perform a Cesarean, or to assist a delivery by other means, in about 3 to 5 per cent of his patients—about one out of every twenty or twenty-five."

"I realize that, Dr. Gordon," Mary assured him, "and I'll trust your judgment completely when the time comes."

"I can see you're going to be a prize patient!" Dr. Gordon gave her a warm smile.

"I have one more question," Mary said. "I've read some things about 'induced labor,' stimulating labor artificially. Is there any advantage to that, or is it dangerous?"

"It can be dangerous, Mary, if unwisely carried out, as in any attempts to 'improve' upon a natural function. Yet it is also a valuable tool in the hands of a skillful physician, when certain circumstances indicate to him that it is necessary.

"Apart from a medical standpoint, however, one reason I hesitate to stimulate labor artificially is that it makes the contractions so much more uncomfortable for the mother. The contractions of an induced labor are not the same as normal contractions; they are stronger, harder, and seem to rise and fall more quickly. The woman in labor has a much more difficult time controlling her relaxation and breathing with these induced contractions, and they may be quite painful. It shortens labor but makes it more distressing for her. Do you have any other questions?"

Mary shook her head, and the doctor rose. "Thanks to your co-operation, you can expect your experience of giving birth to be a safer, shorter, and happier one. I'm looking forward to helping you!"

Mary and John animatedly discussed the information they had gained from the doctor all through supper that evening. Mary began filling the sink with warm water after they had finished, as John cleared the table. Suddenly she cried in dismay,

"John! We forgot all about Mrs. Arkwright! We were supposed to take her home!"

Notes

1. Margaret Hickey, "Too Many Babies Die," *Ladies' Home Journal,* August 1961. Reprinted by special permission of the *Ladies' Home Journal.* Copyright 1961. Curtis Publishing Company.
2. J. Lawrence Cochran, M.D., "Concerning Birth Injuries," *Medical Times,* Vol. 84, 1956, pp. 1336–40.
3. Virginia Larsen, M.D., *Attitudes and Stresses Affecting Perinatal Adjustment* (Fort Steilacoom, Wis.: Mental Health Research Institute, 1966).
4. James Clark Moloney, M.D., "Post-Partum Depression," *Child-Family Digest,* February 1952. (Available from ICEA Supplies Center.)
5. Frederick Schreiber, M.D. "Neurologic Sequaelae of Paranatal Asphyxia," *Journal of Pediatrics,* Vol. 16, 1940, pp. 297–307.
6. A. A. Kawi, M.D., and B. Pasamanick, M.D., *Journal of the American Medical Association,* Vol. 166, 1958, pp. 1420, 1422; A. C. Beck, M.D., and A. H. Rosenthal, M.D., *Obstetric Practice,* 6th ed. (Baltimore: Williams & Wilkins, 1955), p. 1000.
7. T. Berry Brazelton, M.D., "Infant Outcome in Obstetric Anesthesia," *ICEA News,* November-December 1970.

Chapter 9

Bring a Torch, Jeanette, Isabella

*Lo, children are an heritage of the Lord: and
the fruit of the womb is his reward.* Ps. 127:3.

Mary stirred in her sleep, turned restlessly again, and suddenly was
wide awake. There it was! She lay perfectly still, waiting, waiting.
There! Again! Soft as the brush of a butterfly's wing, fragile as a
dewdrop trembling on a leaf, she felt her baby move. A flush of
warm excitement infused her whole being. There it is again! Rising
up on one elbow, she looked to see if John was awake. Watching
him a moment, she was disappointed that he was breathing evenly
in a sound slumber. She hesitated, but couldn't restrain herself
from reaching over and shaking his shoulder gently.

"John," she whispered softly, "wake up! I can feel the baby!
He's moving! John . . ." He mumbled in his sleep and turned over.
She shook him again, a little impatiently this time.

"The baby's moving, John. Wake up, honey!"

" 'Zat so?" he said sleepily. "How nice." He tried to doze off
again, but she was persistent.

"Give me your hand, honey, so you can feel him, too." She took
his hand and placed it over where she'd felt the baby. "Here, put
it right here. Did you feel that? No, no, not there—over here." She
shifted his hand from place to place, but he couldn't feel anything.

"Your hand's always in the wrong place when the baby moves,"
she said, exasperated. "Here—over here now." But it was hopeless.

The baby's movements were too slight for John to detect, so she gave up trying and let him drift back to sleep.

But Mary lay awake, her eyes wide open in the dark, anticipating with delight each delicate flutter of the tiny limbs within her body. A new life inside mine, she thought reverently. Only God could make such a miracle possible! Thank you, God, she whispered to Him softly. He seemed to be standing there beside her, so close, so close, that if she reached out she could touch His hand in the soft darkness of this glad night.

As the first timid rays of the lazy winter sun crept stealthily around the sides and under the hem of Mary's bright yellow and brown kitchen curtains, the aroma of fresh coffee and frying bacon drew John more quickly than usual from his ritual with comb and razor.

"M-m-m-m. Smells good in here. Are we celebrating or something?" He gathered Mary into his arms and gave her an energetic honeymoon hug.

"No," she said, straightening her apron and smoothing down her hair when he let her go, "I just felt like making something special this morning. The biscuits are about done, if you want to sit down." She opened the oven door to take a peek, then closed it for a moment longer while she poured the juice.

"You're not too cross with me for waking you last night, are you, John?" she asked. If he had been cross, he hardly would have remembered it under the spell of the delicious breakfast set on a bright cloth before him, with his radiant young wife beaming at him from across the table.

"Not a bit, honey," he fibbed, as he reached for a biscuit. "You said something about the baby, I remember."

"John!" she scolded. "Don't you remember? The baby was *moving*—first time I've ever felt him. I guess he's sleeping now—I haven't felt even a whisper of a motion this morning." A faraway look came into her eyes as her thoughts turned inward for a moment.

"That's wonderful, Mary," John said. His interest was genuine, now that he was wide awake.

"I was thinking, last night," Mary chatted gaily as he ate, "that I'm not just going to *be* a mother—I already *am* a mother, with a really true baby! Isn't that exciting?"

"Sure is," John agreed, sharing her enthusiasm. "Even though I don't exactly feel like a 'really true' father yet," he teased her, "I like being married to the prettiest 'really true' mother in the whole world!"

Breakfast over, John pulled on his coat and picked up the stack of papers he had graded the night before. Mary still looked so irresistible that he stopped to kiss her again, until she laughingly pushed him away and waved him out the door so he would be on time for his classes.

Mary flew happily through her work that morning. Even the futile efforts of the sun trying to penetrate the sodden clouds didn't dampen her spirits. She finished the breakfast dishes and gave the stove an extra polish before straightening the bedroom and making the bed. As soon as she finished cleaning the front room of their little home, she reached for the second folder the doctor had given her at the office several days before and sat down.

With a new, sobering sense of responsibility, Mary studied its pages again, determined to follow the doctor's instructions conscientiously, for the baby's sake, for John's sake, and for her own.

PRENATAL INSTRUCTIONS

Diet

Maintain a balanced diet of the seven basic foods:
Leafy, green, and yellow vegetables
Citrus fruit, tomatoes, raw greens
Potatoes, vegetables, fruits
Milk, cheese, ice cream
Meat, poultry, fish, eggs
Bread, flour, cereals
Butter and margarine
Limit the weight gain to fifteen to twenty pounds by moderate eating habits.

Eat a little less than usual, especially sweets and starchy foods.

Do not skip meals, or go on crash diets to avoid weight gain as many pregnant women foolishly do.

Drink several glasses of water daily.

Use salt sparingly during both pregnancy and nursing.

Avoid overeating at any one meal during the last two months of pregnancy.

A vitamin supplement may be prescribed for you.

Relaxation

After the fifth month of pregnancy (before, if you wish) relax in the following "three-quarter" position:

> Lie on your left side, your head and right shoulder resting on a pillow.
>
> Put the left arm behind you, curved slightly at the elbow, and bend the left knee.
>
> Draw the right knee partway up, toward your chest.
>
> Place a pillow under the right knee so that your abdomen barely touches the floor or the bed.
>
> If you are not comfortable, try a larger or smaller pillow under the right knee.
>
> Be sure to have none of your weight on your abdomen. It wouldn't hurt the baby, but would be less comfortable for you.
>
> Keep your abdomen sagging limply beneath you like a hammock. Use this position for sleep at night, also during the later months of pregnancy. (See Fig. 4.)

Later in pregnancy, in addition to the left-side position, practice relaxing in the "reclining-chair" or "lounge-chair" position, with the chair back at a 45° angle, the knees resting on supports, and pillows or arm rests under the arms. (See Fig. 9.) If you don't have a reclining chair, turn a straight-back chair upside down on the floor, place pillows against its back, and lean against that, with pillows or rolled blankets for support under your knees and arms. When comfortable, allow all muscles to become completely limp, and do not move for twenty minutes. Then get up slowly, as before.

Exercises

I. *Muscular control of the vagina and perineum.*

This exercise is *very important*. Tighten all the muscles of the pelvic floor (including urethra, vagina, and anus) by drawing them in as one would clench a fist.

Hold these muscles tightly for a count of three.

Slowly, slowly, "let go" until the muscles are completely slack.

Do this twelve to twenty times in a row, at least twice each day.

II. *Stretching the leg muscles inside the upper thigh.*

Lie on your back, bend the knees, keeping feet flat on the floor, and move your heels halfway back toward the hips.

Let your knees fall widely apart.

Stretch them in an effort to touch the floor on each side.

Bring your knees together, then let them fall outward again.

Do this several times each day. (See Fig. 5.)

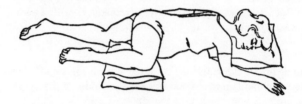

Fig. 4. Lateral, or three-quarter position for relaxation. It is essential that the right knee and thigh be supported in a raised position so that there will be no weight or pressure on the abdomen. The abdomen should sag limply below the body in complete relaxation.

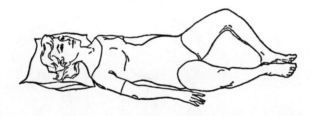

Fig. 5. Stretching the inner thigh muscles. Try to touch the floor on each side with the knees simultaneously (you won't make it, but come as close as you can). This exercise strengthens the inner leg muscles so that they will not become tired during the second stage of labor when the legs are in this position for some time.

III. *Loosening the joints of the lower spine and pelvis.*

 A. Pelvic rock.

   To prevent or relieve backache, get down on hands and knees.

     First, arch your back like an angry cat, putting your head down between your arms, which are kept straight at the elbow. Tighten the muscles of the buttocks, upper legs and pelvic floor. (See Fig. 6.)

     Second, raise your head high, and let your back sag like the overstretched seat of a canvas chair. (See Fig. 7.)

 B. Squatting.

   Sit on your heels, knees wide apart, like a primitive woman.

     Lean against a wall for balance, if necessary. (See Fig. 1.)

   Sit "Indian style" or tailor style" frequently, with knees out, feet crossed, and drawn up close to the body.

IV. *Practicing good posture.*

   Stand against a door and try to touch it with the small of your back.

   Place your hands under your ribs on each side of the chest.

   Now pretend you are lifting the rib cage *up.*

   As you do this, you will automatically straighten your shoulders, tuck your hips under, and raise your chin.

   Take a walk each day, using this good posture. (Be careful to avoid chilling, or becoming overtired.)

   Hold your head high as if proud to be pregnant. You *are* proud, aren't you?

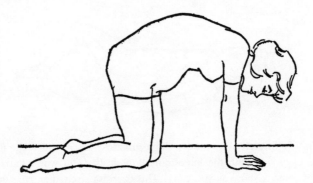

Fig. 6. Pelvic rocking, exercise III A, position 1. This limbers the pelvic joints and also strengthens the back muscles.

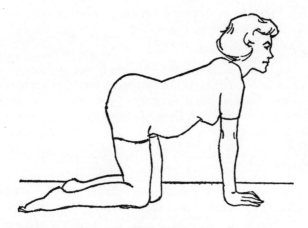

Fig. 7. Pelvic rocking, position 2.

Breathing

There are three types of breathing to recognize and learn to control.

I. *"Sleep" breathing.*

The muscles of the abdomen and lower chest rise and fall gently when this is done properly, as in sleep.

Take a breath deep into the diaphragm.

Hold for a count of three, then exhale slowly.

Relax more completely with each exhalation.

II. *"Work" breathing.*

Expand the chest and diaphragm while taking deeper, faster breaths. Use this breathing during any activity to help avoid shortness of breath and fatigue. Be sure to breathe *out* completely after each breath that is drawn in.

III. *Breath holding.*

Take a full, deep breath. Exhale, blowing out until the chest seems completely empty. Take another breath, drawing it in deeply and hold it—for a count of ten, fifteen, twenty. Gradually lengthen the time the breath can be held comfortably. Exhale slowly, not suddenly, after holding the breath. Take a "cleansing breath" once or twice, deeply in and out, before trying to hold the breath again.

This is the breathing used while bearing down to push the baby out. Remember always to take a cleansing breath in and out before and after breath holding.

IV. *Panting.*

Breathe rapidly with little short breaths in the upper chest, mouth open. You will be asked to do this only when you must not bear down, as during the final moments of the baby's birth, so his head will emerge slowly and you will not tear. Concentrate on breathing *out*: "a—HU, a—HU, a—HU."

SUMMARY

Drink enough water, eat small, well-balanced meals, use little salt. Set aside thirty minutes each day, *faithfully to do the following*:

Lie on back, practice slow, deep breathing for three or four minutes.

Turn onto left side, slip pillow under left knee and thigh and relax *completely* for twenty minutes.

Before getting up, turn on back, practice stretching inner leg muscles a few times (Exercise II).

Get onto hands and knees, arch and lower back a few times (Exercise III A).

Stand up slowly. Practice breath holding.

Use "work" breathing to begin tasks around the house.

Practice vaginal exercise frequently, while sitting, standing, or lying down.

Sit "Indian style" while watching TV, reading, et cetera.

Practice "squatting" while dusting furniture or "picking up."

Practice good posture and diaphragm breathing during a daily walk.

Mary finished reading the folder, put it down on the floor open at the summary, and lay down on her back. She practiced the slow, deep-sleep breathing ten times, and then turned over to relax, but found she had no pillow for her knee.

Getting up again, she chose three flexible pillows—one for her head, and two to experiment with, to find which was the more comfortable, for her right knee and thigh. She chose the smaller one, as her abdomen was still fairly small. She lay down and let her whole body sag.

The first few minutes she felt restless, but did not move, taking deep, lazy "sleeping" breaths. Eventually she became completely relaxed, and was floating off on a pink cloud somewhere when she heard the mailman come up the hall and drop some mail in their box. She did not flicker an eyelash, however, or stir a muscle until the timer on her kitchen clock signaled that her time was up.

Then she turned on her back, drew up her knees, and practiced dropping them to the outside simultaneously. She did this only four or five times, as it really made the muscles "pull" on the inside of her thighs, showing how weak these muscles were.

Before getting up, she got onto her hands and knees and alternately arched and dropped her back half a dozen times. Then, tremendously pleased with her own self-control at not having jumped up at once to get the mail—although she had been tempted—she got up slowly and walked out into the hall.

There was a letter from Aunt Em, and Mary sat down to read it:

December 5

Dear John and Mary,

We have thought of you both so many times since you visited us last summer, and have prayed that God would bless your lives together as He has blessed ours.

George had a slight stroke the day after Thanksgiving. He has had a bit of paralysis on his left side since then, but we are grateful that he has no other aftereffects.

As the Christmas season approaches, we trust it will be a most blessed time for you—your first Christmas together. May God fill you with a realization of the beauty and joy of the event of that first Christmas time—the birth of our Saviour and Lord.

With love,
Aunt Emma

The evergreens in yard after yard put on their only blossoms of the year—shiny red, blue, yellow, pink and gold lights, as the heightened anticipation of another Christmas grew keener. Day after day the little town increased its adorning to celebrate the birth of the Christ child. Silver bells and streamers framed the streets. Passers-by greeted one another gaily and hummed along with the age-old carols echoing from the stores along the avenue. Even nature co-operated in the festivities, silently adding delicate white trimming to shrubs and treetops, houses, lawns, and fences.

It seemed to Mary that there had never been a lovelier Advent season. Her thoughts turned again and again to another Mary, with an affinity she had never felt before. The maiden of old trusted God and obeyed Him, Mary thought to herself, but how she must have been misunderstood and ridiculed by friends and relatives for her condition. How hard it must have been to be pregnant and not married—beginning to look big, as I am, and not have anyone understand. I wonder if her own mother believed her. How could she explain—"Mother, I am pregnant, but it is God Who made me so. You see, an angel came and told me how it would be. . . ."

No one would believe her! And how could she explain to Joseph, her beloved? Mary felt in her own soul the agony of misunderstanding experienced by that other Mary, whose growing body could no longer conceal the secret of her heart. No wonder she had rushed to Elizabeth, to a woman who walked with God, who would listen and believe her story.

What did Elizabeth say to her? Such happy words. "Blessed art thou among women," she had proclaimed, "and blessed is the fruit of thy womb."

The "fruit of the womb"—how often that lovely phrase is used in the Bible of a tiny baby like mine, Mary realized. Christ, too, before His birth, was called the "fruit of the womb"—a "fruit" like my own child. Jesus could have come some other way, as Adam had. But He chose instead to come to live on earth by way of a woman's body. No wonder Mary's heart overflowed with joy at Elizabeth's words, as she sang in reply,

My soul doth magnify the Lord,
And my spirit hath rejoiced in God my Saviour. . . .
For He that is mighty hath done to me great things;
And holy is His name. . . .

"Are you quite sure you don't want to go along, Mary?" her mother asked, as the carolers prepared to leave the Johnsons' on Christmas Eve.

"No, Mother. You need my help if the carolers are all coming here afterward. Jo Lynn can show John all the places that we usually stop to carol."

"You sure you don't mind, Mary?" Jo Lynn asked in surprise.

"Not a bit!" Mary replied. "Have a good time now."

John and Mary exchanged a secret glance that said more than any words of devotion ever spoken. She blew him a kiss as he and Jo Lynn went out the door. She felt a growing security in John's love, a bond that drew them closer with every passing day. Jo Lynn is so young, so ignorant of life, Mary thought smugly to herself. How could I ever have been jealous of her?

Mrs. Johnson had not failed to notice her daughter's new poise. She realized that if Mary had not always been so sensitive, Jo Lynn wouldn't have been such a tease. She began slicing the nut bread, and Mary spread the softened butter on each slice before arranging them in even rows on the bread tray. While they worked, she told her mother some of the things she had been learning and how much she looked forward to having her baby naturally, because she believed that God meant giving birth to be a blessed experience for a mother.

Mrs. Johnson thought back to her own experiences, but the memories were so unpleasant that she deliberately turned her attention to something else. She was worried about Mary's idealism. She knew from sad experience that giving birth simply wasn't like that. How hard it was going to be for her to see her daughter disappointed. But Mary seemed so confident, so happy—she decided it was better to keep her doubts to herself.

Mr. Johnson had started a crackling fire to warm the numb feet and hands of the carolers when they returned. The fragrant cocoa was steaming on the stove, and the table was laden with Christmas Eve delicacies when the first stray notes of "Hark, the Herald Angels Sing" reached their ears from far down the street.

"Here they come!" exclaimed Mary happily, moving near the window to hear more clearly. She stood just behind the living-room draperies where she could not be seen, as the carolers sang their last refrain before streaming up onto the porch and into the cheerful hospitality of the Johnsons' home:

> Bring a torch, Jeannette, Isabella,
>   Bring a torch, it is dark in the stall;
> Jesus awaits, good folks of the village,
>   Run quickly, I hear Mary's soft call,
> Ah!—Ah!—Beautiful is the mother,
>   Ah!—Ah!—Beautiful is her child!

Chapter 10

Words of Life and Beauty

Open thou mine eyes, that I may behold
wondrous things out of thy law. Ps. 119:18.

Several weeks elapsed before John and Mary were able to meet with the pastor to discuss childbirth and the Bible again. John hurried over to the parsonage one Friday evening after an early basketball game. Mary was already there as she had spent the afternoon with Mrs. Dirkson.

Pastor Dirkson invited them into his study, where his reference material was readily available. He seated himself at his desk after the others had made themselves comfortable, arranged some notes on the desk before him, and leaned back in his chair.

"Let's review, first of all, the two passages that we discussed last time," he suggested. "What does the Genesis passage teach us about motherhood?"

"Well, I'd say," John began, since the women didn't answer, "that it teaches that we don't accomplish anything in this life without giving something of ourselves in return. In other words, Eve was to renounce herself—give of her own strength, in her efforts to bring forth a child."

"That's true," Mrs. Dirkson interrupted earnestly, "but the Bible says that Eve recognized her children as coming from God, and she doesn't say *anything* about toiling in birth."

"Wasn't Eve punished for her sin at all then?" Mary asked.

"I've always thought," Mrs. Dirkson replied, "that Eve first fully realized the awful consequences of her sin, and must have suffered an agony of remorse when she witnessed one son slain and her first-born son the murderer!"

"Do you remember how God *comforted* her?" her husband asked.

"Yes, Carl. God gave her the privilege of giving birth again! I've often seen, in my mind, the warm, sweet body of little Seth nestled in Eve's arms, as she kissed him over and over through her tears of repentance and grief. She tells us herself that God sent her this little baby to comfort her heart because of Abel's death."

"Then could it possibly be," Mary suggested thoughtfully, "that Genesis 3:16 means that Eve was to be disciplined by giving of herself through all the years of her life rather than just by the one discipline of giving birth?"

"I believe so, Mary," the pastor told her, "for, you see, Adam's 'renunciation' wasn't that of a day but of a lifetime. Paul tells us in I Timothy 2:15 that all Christian women, like Eve, should work out their salvation 'through *motherhood,* if only women *continue* in faith, love and holiness, with a sober mind.'[1]

"The key word in Paul's statement is *continue.* This is a *going-on* process in a woman's life. She's to continue to give of herself in all the Christian graces, especially as an example before the eyes of her children.

"Rabbi Hirsch shows how the Jews believed that Genesis 3:16 applies to a woman's whole life, for he says:

> Of the 'renunciation' of the man, the wife is, to the greatest part free. Not by the sweat of her brow has she to gain her bread. . . . The whole life of a woman, from earliest girlhood, is a life of sacrifice, giving herself up for others. . . . There is no higher happiness for a woman than to have children."[2]

"Well, of course!" Mary noted. "Almost every girl wants to get married some day and spend her life raising a family."

Pastor Dirkson nodded in agreement. "Yes, Mary. But now, what does the passage in John teach us about the mother?"

"Hey, here's an interesting thing!" John exclaimed, as a thought struck him. "The verse in John sort of compliments the one in Genesis, doesn't it? Genesis 3:16 tells only of a mother's sorrow of renunciation, but Jesus goes beyond this to tell of a mother's great *joy,* the reward of her efforts, especially just after she's given of herself in childbirth."

"It's true of a mother then, isn't it," Pastor Dirkson said smiling, "that she finds it 'more blessed to give than to receive'? But we must go on.

"Apart from the verses we've just discussed, all the others about childbirth in the Bible fall into two categories. First, there are specific instances of women in the Hebrew culture giving birth, and, second, there are illustrations of some aspect of the birth of a child that were used by the prophets and Paul in teaching the people.

"Unfortunately, several of these passages have been so distorted in our English translations that they give very *in*accurate pictures of the childbirth customs of the ancient Hebrew women in their more primitive, more Oriental culture. Do you remember what we said their attitude toward birth was?"

"The most important thing," Mrs. Dirkson suggested, "was their belief that a mother was blessed by God if He gave her the privilege of giving birth to, and of nursing, her own babies. She was considered 'cursed' only if she didn't have children."

"This is most important, Ruth," her husband said. "The Jews thought so highly of motherhood that Jerusalem itself was compared to a mother who comforts her babies, who carries them on her side, and bounces them happily on her knees. So any translations involving the birth of a child, must fit into this cultural belief that it was a blessing to the mother.

"To show you how some of these verses have been mistranslated, let me explain what the Hebrew and Greek words for childbirth are. There are five of these words, all of which, when applied to a birth, mean simply 'bringing forth,' or 'begetting,' or 'making,' and so forth. Frequently, however, we find these words mistranslated as 'travail,' 'sorrow,' 'pain,' 'pangs,' and in the newer translations, even as 'writhe'!

"These Bible words are *yalad* and *chul,* in the Old Testament, and *tiktō, gennaō,* and *ōdinō,* in the New Testament. We'll discuss these five words one at a time.

"*Yalad,* for example, is used, not only of a mother giving birth, but also of a *father* having sons 'born' to him, as Isaac was '*born* **(yalad)** to Abraham,' and as sons were '*born* **(yalad)** to Jacob.' *Yalad* is used of fathers in this way dozens of times in the genealogies: this man *begat* **(yalad)** a son, and he begat **(yalad)** a son, and so forth.

"*Yalad* is even used sometimes of God's acts in creation, as when He says to Job:

> Knowest thou . . . who hath *begotten* **(yalad)** the drops of dew?

"It is only when *yalad* is used of a woman that it is ever translated as '*travail.*' "

John was obviously disturbed. "This is more unfair than what was done to *etsev!*" he exploded. "It doesn't seem to have any justification at all!"

"It has no justification from a linguistic standpoint," the pastor told him. "But look now at what has been done to the second Hebrew word for giving birth, *chul.* Do you remember the Hebrew fondness for parallelism—how they liked to have two words meaning essentially the same thing, so they could use them in parallel phrases? They used *yalad* and *chul* interchangeably in this way.

"Not only is *chul* used of a mother, but it is also used of God's part in a birth, and in His creating of all things. He is spoken of as '*shaping* **(chul)**' the unborn child in the womb, or of 'making the hinds to *calve* **(chul)**,' or as '*making* **(chul)**' a man, or as '*forming* **(chul)**' the earth. *Chul* and *yalad* are sometimes used interchangeably of God's acts of creation, as in this verse found in Deuteronomy 32:18.

> Of the Rock that *begat* **(yalad)** thee thou are unmindful, and hast forgotten God that *formed* **(chul)** thee."

"If these words are used interchangeably of God, can you give us an example of their being used for a mother, too?" John asked. "Indeed I can," Pastor Dirkson replied. "How about this passage from Micah 4:9, 10, in the Revised Standard Version?

> . . . *pangs* **(chul)** have seized you like a woman in *travail* **(yalad)**.
>
> *Writhe* **(chul)** and groan, O daughter of Zion, like a woman in *travail* **(yalad)**."

John shifted angrily in his chair, but Pastor Dirkson reminded him that mistranslations such as this were unintentional. They were mistakes, made because the translators had been blinded by their own culture.

"Let's look at these New Testament words for childbirth now," he suggested, after John had calmed down. "As I mentioned before, these words are *tiktō, gennaō,* and *ōdinō*. All three of these words are used interchangeably of childbirth, all three are used at one time or another in the Septuagint to translate *yalad,* and all three are used to translate *chul*. This shows how closely all five of these words are interrelated.

"We discussed *tiktō* in connection with John 16:21 last time. It is occasionally mistranslated as 'travail,' but it is usually translated correctly as 'to bring forth' a child.

"*Gennaō* is used of a mother giving birth, or of a father 'begetting,' as was *yalad*. In the genealogies of Matthew 1, for example, *gennaō* is used of the father begetting a son, over and over. It is also a word used of God as a parent, as were *yalad* and *chul*. For instance in Hebrews 1:5:

> For unto which of the angels said he at any time. Thou art my Son, this day have I *begotten* **(gennaō)** thee?

"The fifth word used of childbirth, *ōdinō,* is the New Testament word most often mistranslated as the 'pain' or 'travail' of a mother. But we know this isn't correct, because it is used interchangeably with the other words for childbirth, and, also, because the early

Christians translated it into Latin as *parturio,* from which we get our English word 'parturition,' which simply refers to the *process* of giving birth. *Ōdinō* is best translated as 'labor,' *i.e.,* the *act* of bringing to birth, as Paul says,

> My little children, of whom I *labor* (**ōdinō**) in birth again, until Christ be formed in you. (Gal. 4:19.)

"Now this isn't to say," Pastor Dirkson explained, "that pain wasn't ever present in a birth in Bible days. For example, we might say, 'Janet had a baby yesterday.' We're making a simple statement of fact—as these Hebrew and Greek words do—we're not explaining what *kind* of a birth experience Janet had.

"In the few times in the Bible in which it mentions that difficulty arose for a woman giving birth, *additional* words are used to make this fact clear. And, in every case, these additional words make it clear that the mother is suffering from exhaustion—from not being able to *work* any longer, as it says in Isaiah 37:3:

> The children are brought to the birth, and there is not *strength* to bring forth.

"This confirms our belief that the ancient Hebrews thought of childbirth primarily as a 'work' process. Let's look at the story of Rachel, for an example. Here a word is added to show that her labor was 'stiff, difficult, fierce' when Benjamin was born."

"Rachel died in childbirth, didn't she?" Mary asked.

"Yes, Mary. But remember that Rachel had wanted children. In fact, she was so jealous of her sister Leah's having children that one can almost see her stamp her foot as she demands of Jacob petulantly,

" 'Give me children, or else I die!'

"God heard her prayer when she turned to Him and gave her a son. At Joseph's birth she was so delighted that she cried, 'Oh, God! Give to me *another* son!" (RSV.) Notice that this was a *request* Rachel made.

"But with Rachel's second labor all wasn't well. She couldn't have known beforehand that her *second* child would be born with much greater toil than the first. Something was obviously wrong, for the midwife tells her before the child's birth,

" 'This one, too, is a *son* for you.'

"Since the midwife was aware of the sex of the child before his birth, he was obviously in an *abnormal* position, and Rachel toiled in vain to give birth to him, until she was weeping and exhausted. As she felt the last shreds of her energy slipping away, and her child not yet born, the midwife tries to encourage her by saying, 'Come now, Rachel, don't be afraid. Push just a little more, and we'll have this boy delivered, too.'

"Rachel succeeded in giving Benjamin birth, but she was too weakened to recover and she died. I wonder if you realize that Rachel's is the only death caused by childbirth that's recorded in the entire Bible?"

"Why, no," John said. "I thought there were many."

Pastor Dirkson explained, shaking his head, "One other death at childbirth is recorded, but it wasn't caused from the birth itself, but from the shock of bad news occurring right at this time. And this mother, too, died after the birth of her *second* child. (I Sam. 4:21; 14:3.) Do you remember the story of Eli?"

"Wasn't he the high priest when Hannah brought her boy Samuel to the temple?" Mary asked.

"Yes. He was a godly man, but his sons were wicked, and on one occasion they took the ark of God with them into battle. The ark was stolen by the Philistines. Eli's sons were killed in battle, and when Eli heard the news, he fell over in his chair, and died of a broken neck.

"Eli's daughter-in-law was pregnant, and when this evil news was brought to her, her labor began prematurely, at seven months, according to Jewish tradition. The Bible relates that she didn't even know when her child had been born because she was so absorbed with her grief.

"The midwives tried to get her attention and to comfort her by saying, 'Look! Look here! Your child has already been born.

You have another little son! Look!' But 'she answered them not, neither did she regard it.' And she died of grief, sobbing over and over,

> The ark of God is taken!
> The glory is departed from Israel!
> The ark of God is taken!"

"This surely opens my eyes to some things, pastor," John said. "I've always thought of childbirth in the Bible as being associated with pain, death, or woe."

"Many of us, John," the pastor said, "have been as guilty of misinterpreting passages about childbirth through careless reading, as translators have been. Childbirth in the Bible is primarily spoken of as a beautiful event, even in our English Bibles, but we've somehow overlooked this fact. And in all the actual records of a birth, apart from the two we just mentioned, the association is a happy one. The mothers often seem especially aware of God at this time and of His great goodness to them.

"We can still interpret correctly the examples of childbirth used for illustration by the prophets and by Paul, even when they're inaccurately translated. Remember that the comparison isn't 'pain,' or 'anguish,' in every case, as the English indicates, but look for the phenomenon, or *aspect* of a birth experience in the Hebrew culture that is being used for comparison.

"Is it, for example, the groan or gasp of effort that accompanies the work of bearing down? Is it the posture—crouching or kneeling and bending over the abdomen, as if aiding a contraction? Is it absorption in the task, so that one neither sees nor hears what is going on around him? Is it the fact that birth occurs when it is unexpected, or is it the certainty that a woman with a child in her womb must some day give birth to him? and so on.

"Some of these comparisons are unhappy ones. In Jeremiah, the prophet of the leisure classes of court society, for example, we find examples of gasping, being out of breath, or of hands so weak from the labor of birth that they can no longer grasp a support. You see, the Bible reveals people as they were. And although most Hebrew women seem to have had normal birth experiences, a few did not, which is true in any culture."

"What I'd like to know," John mused, "is how this idea of a curse of 'pain' on Eve came to be believed at all, if it's not anywhere in the Bible, or even in the early theology of the Jews."

"I'd be glad to show you some of the ways this concept developed," Pastor Dirkson offered, "if you'd care to come back next week."

"I'd surely like to," John replied. "Wouldn't you, Mary?" She nodded, so he suggested, "How about Thursday night? We have a late game next Friday, so I couldn't make it then."

Mrs. Dirkson explained that special choir rehearsals for the Easter cantata were to begin the following Thursday, but that they were welcome to come afterward, and all agreed.

Notes

1. I Timothy 2:15, The New English Bible (New York: Oxford University Press and Cambridge University Press, 1961).
2. Rabbi Samson Raphael Hirsch, *The Pentateuch* (a translation and commentary), Vol. I, Genesis, rendered into English by the publisher (London: Isaac Levy, 1959), p. 83.

Chapter 11

Through a Glass, Darkly

At present all I know is a little fraction of the truth, but the time will come when I shall know it as fully as God now knows me! I Cor. 13:12 (Phillips translation.)

Mary put away the last of the pots and pans, and wiped up the remaining traces of flour. She could never manage to bake, it seemed, without getting flour from ceiling to floor. She hoped John would be pleased with her pie. Of course, the filling had burned a bit before she poured it into the crust—but maybe he wouldn't notice.

She stepped back to take one last critical look at her handiwork before quickly mixing up a hot dish to pop into the oven. There wasn't time left for anything else. She slipped into the bedroom to brighten her weary features before John came home.

"Hi! Anybody home?" he called cheerily as he came in the door. Mary laid down her brush and went to greet him. He came up beside her, where he could reach around her for a quick hug, and she tipped her head obligingly so he could kiss her.

As they sat together over their evening meal, John related the events of the day. Mary was unusually tired, so she said little. After John had finished his dinner, Mary served him his pie and coffee, and took her place again, folding her napkin carefully over and over in her lap, as she waited expectantly for his comment.

John finished his pie, looked up, and asked, "Mary, may I please

106

have another cup of coffee?" To his astonishment, she rose abruptly from her chair, burst into tears, and flung herself out of the room. Bewildered, he got up from the table and followed her.

"Honey, whatever is the matter?" he asked anxiously. "Did I say or do something to hurt you?"

"No," she sobbed, "it's just—here I slaved all afternoon because you've been wanting a pie like Aunt Em's, and then," she daubed at her eyes, "you don't even say *one word* about it!" She burst into a fresh flood of tears again, feeling sheepish over her emotion but unable to control it.

John thought to himself that the pie wasn't exactly like one of Aunt Em's, but he knew better than to say so!

"Mary," he tried to console her, "I'm an ungrateful wretch, and I'm terribly sorry. It was thoughtful of you to take so much time to please me, and I love you for it. Forgive me, honey? Remember what Uncle George said about the two bears?"

Mary was quieter now, listening.

"Bear, and forbear," John said softly. "I'll try to bear your burdens—share them with you more, honey, if you'll forbear this time and forgive me for being thoughtless?"

Mary nodded, her head against his shoulder. Suddenly a thought occurred to John. "Mary," he asked, "did you do your relaxing today?" She shook her head.

"Yesterday?" She shook her head again.

"The day before?"

"No," she admitted sheepishly.

"Now look, Mary," he said, his voice rising, "I'd rather have you take care of your own health and our baby's than to go fussing over me!"

"But . . ." She tried to explain, but he interrupted her excuses.

"You know what Dr. Gordon said—that most women in our society are too tense, and that if you want a comfortable birth you won't have it just by wishing for it! Remember that he said it would be safer for you and the baby, too, if you'd do as he said."

Mary listened abjectively as he lectured on in locker-room enthusiasm.

"When I take my boys out for spring training, I say to them, 'Any of you guys can get out there and run, see? But that's not enough for me! I want you to do your best *every day* in obeying the training rules. *Understand?* You won't win the race on the day of the meet but in all the weeks of patient training and discipline that come beforehand. *Understand?*'

"It's the same with you, Mary. Any mother can give birth, but that's not enough! Because I love you, I want you to have the happiest, safest, and best possible experience, and I want you to be as faithful in training for it as I expect my boys to be in training for a meet!"

"*Understand?*" Mary mimicked him, smiling now. "All right, preacher. I promise."

"Take time to be yourself, too, honey, and don't worry so much about me," John added. "Why don't you go in and relax right now before we go over to the Dirksons'? I'll call you when time's up."

Mary took her two pillows and lay down on the living-room floor to relax. Because she'd been upset, it took her nearly five minutes to let her whole body become limp. But because she had learned to relax well, in spite of several days' lapse, she was soon able to release all her physical and emotional tensions. Shortly after she became relaxed, she fell asleep, since she was exhausted. It seemed as if only a few minutes had elapsed before John was shaking her gently, saying it was time for them to get ready to go.

"Tonight," Pastor Dirkson began, as they sat in his study once more, "as we discuss this subject for the last time, I'll attempt to show you how this evil teaching that God damned all married women with pain developed. We've already seen that this teaching isn't Biblical and that it isn't a part of Jewish theology. Some of our theologians have thought that it was carried over into the Church from the tradition of the Pharisees, but this isn't true. In fact, because the Jews have never believed that God wants women to suffer pain in childbirth, they haven't hesitated to relieve this pain whenever it *has* occurred, as far as their knowledge has made this possible. One present-day rabbi says:

In rabbinic writings the question is never raised [*i.e.*, of refusing to relieve pain in childbirth]; as has been remarked, 'the prohibition of analgesics would contradict Jewish theology.' Indeed, the sympathy of Jewish law for the sufferings accompanying childbirth is so strong that some of its leading exponents justify the recourse to contraceptive sterilization by mothers who fear the pain of further births."[1]

"But Christians don't oppose the use of analgesics either," John pointed out.

"Not today," the pastor explained, "but the Church strongly opposed the relief of pain in childbirth in the last century, because they taught that a woman's cries and screams of pain in childbirth pleased the ears of God! Did you know, for example, that in France two women were burned to death by the Church,[2]—the one for accepting relief for her pain in childbirth, and the other for giving it to her?"

"How perfectly awful!" Mary gasped.

"But during the same period in which these two women were martyred by the Church, a great deal was being done to reduce man's struggle with his 'curse' of tilling the ground, with the development of the tools and machinery of the industrial age. The Church was completely inconsistent in this. They saw no reason to oppose the development of labor-saving devices, on the grounds that it would thwart God's punishment of 'toil' on man, and interfere with stalwart Christian character. But of the woman, it was declared that any relief of pain in childbirth was completely unjustifiable, because God had decreed that she should suffer. These Church leaders said . . ." Pastor Dirkson paused, opened a book on his desk to a passage he had marked, and read:

Let . . . our women be trained to have courage and resilience, and to the proper appreciation of their high vocation and duties; then I guarantee that they will not cry out for chloroform under the pangs of labor, but cling with redoubled love and sacrifice to the beings whom they bring into existence in pain.[3]

"But why should it be more important for women to endure suffering than for men?" John asked. "I don't understand this."

"I'll show you in a moment, John, how women were singled out as needing special punishment from God. Actually, the whole concept of physical pain making a person more godly was widely believed in one period of Church history—so much so, that pain was frequently self-inflicted, in order to make oneself 'holy.' The body was regarded as intrinsically evil and needing to be 'mortified,' as the flagellants did when they whipped themselves.

"Here again the Church teaching differed from the Jews,' which never suggested that 'there is virtue or some desirable *beau ideal* in bodily anguish.'[4] And of course, this is also a distortion of the New Testament teaching that Christians may have to endure sufferings because of their faith but that God will bring blessing in spite of, and during, these sufferings of persecution by others.

"This idea of physical pain leading to godliness continued to be applied to married women, even though no longer applied to men, until very recently.

"But let's go back now to the origin of Christianity and see if we can spot where this teaching began. In the first-century Church there is no evidence that women were singled out for a special curse. As a matter of fact, early Christians write in most lofty terms of the parturient Christian woman.

"A second-century Christian, Clement of Alexandria, tells us that motherhood is such an exalted state that it can be compared to the motherhood of the Church over the believers.[5] And he compares the milk of a nursing mother, which he says is given to her for her infant by God, to the heavenly 'manna, the celestial food of angels that flowed down from heaven on the ancient Hebrews.'[6]

"Still another early Christian demonstrates that God doesn't inflict pain on mankind and that a Christian need not abuse his physical body by pain in order to become godly, for he says:

What is pain but the interruption of harmony?
. . . There is therefore no pain where there is harmony."[7]

"He sounds like a twentieth-century Christian," John observed. "Remember our discussion about the causes for suffering, Mary?" Mary smiled that she did indeed remember.

Pastor Dirkson opened another of the volumes on the desk in front of him. "After the beginning of the third century A.D.," he said, "one finds a change of attitude beginning among Christians— a change which degrades womanhood, looks on the intercourse of marriage as sinful lust, on motherhood as a necessary evil, and on the birth of a child as the shameful consequence of sin. With such a degrading attitude toward women, the idea that God had singled her out for special punishment began to form. The first expression of this attitude is found in the following passage." He pulled the open volume closer, and began to read:

> No one of you at all, best beloved sisters, from the time that she had first known the Lord, and learned the truth concerning her own (that is, woman's) condition, would have desired too gladsome a style of dress; so as not rather to go about in humble garb, and to effect meanness of appearance, walking about as Eve mourning and repentant, in order that by every garb of penitence she might the more fully expiate that which she derives from Eve. . . . And do you know that you are each an Eve? The sentence of God on this sex of yours lives in this age: the guilt must of necessity live too. *You* are the devil's gateway: *you* are the unsealer of that forbidden tree: *you* are the first deserter of the divine law: *you* are she who persuaded him whom the devil was not valiant enough to attack. *You* destroyed so easily God's image, man. On account of *your* desert, that is, death—even the Son of God had to die![8]

Mary shuddered. "I can almost feel the long, bony finger of that old man pointing at me now!"

Pastor Dirkson turned a few more pages of his book. "This same writer," he said, "tells us that the birth of children is the evil result of marriage and that marriage is in the same class as fornication and adultery. He says that the curse of 'Sodom and Gomorrah' will fall with 'woe' upon the woman who commits the sin of marrying and that God will punish her with 'the burdensome fruit of marriage heaving in the womb, [or] in the bosom.' "⁹

"This is incredible!" John exclaimed, interrupting.

"Adam's punishment is no longer mentioned side by side with Eve's as in Jewish and early Christian writings. A woman now stands alone, as an inferior, ignoble creature, created for man's downfall, punished by 'the sorrows and the groans of women'[10] and by being her husband's slave, if she marries. By twisting Biblical truths, these Church leaders taught that married women were under a special curse, and that only the virgin could escape the 'curse of Eve.' Not only that, but they taught that a woman who did *not* marry was *no longer inferior to man!* They said, '. . . with that of men your lot and your condition is equal.'[11] They even went so far as to say:

> Virginity has no children, but what is more, it has contempt for offspring. . . ."[12]

"How could anyone think of a tiny baby as *contemptible!*" Mary protested.

Pastor Dirkson shook his head. "Of course," he added, "this was also a twisting of the early Church's teaching that virginity, for a man or a woman, was a holy calling—one of 'standing constantly before God' as His special servant. The right motive makes a great difference! By the fourth century, Mary, there were even mothers who deserted their own children to attempt to prove their holiness![13] This is completely contrary to New Testament teaching, and completely contrary to Jewish teaching. In fact, the rabbi who has a large family has always been regarded with great respect. *Not* to marry was regarded by the Jews in centuries past as a sin. The Talmud states that the man who remains unmarried 'is not even a Man,'[14] and that—" The pastor shuffled through his notes, looking for the quotation he wanted. "Here it is:

> If a man remain unmarried after the age of twenty, his life is a constant transgression. The Holy One—Blessed be He!—waits until that period to see if one enters the matrimonial state, and curses his bones if he remain single.[15]

"During the Reformation there was a reaction to the Church's teachings about marriage. We find pastors of that time marrying, but the change in attitude was only partial. Married women still occupied a lowly position in the social order. In fact, in the Thomas Matthew Bible of A.D. 1537, husbands are even advised to beat their wives if necessary! He based this on the teaching of I Peter 3:3:

> Sara obeyed Abraham and called hym Lorde, whose daughters ye are as longe as ye doe well and be not afraid of every shadowe.

"Down at the bottom of the page we find this inspirational footnote:

> He dwelleth wyth his wyfe according to knowledge, that taketh her as a necessarye healper and not as a bond slave. And yf she be not obedient, and helpful unto him endevoureth to beate the feare of God into her heade, that thereby she maye be compelled to learne the dutie and to do it."

"It sounds as though Sir Thomas Matthew must have had a difficult wife," John laughed, shaking his head. "I wonder if his drastic treatment worked."

"Better not try it," Mary warned him, smiling.

"Not only did women have a low position in society," Pastor Dirkson said, "but it was not until *this* time—during the sixteenth and seventeenth centuries—that the concept of 'pain in childbirth' was included in the 'curse of Eve' teaching. Previously only the 'sorrow' and 'groans of toil' in childbirth, the 'sorrow' of the bereavement of children, and subjection to one's husband were mentioned.

"For example, according to German scholars, the word most often associated with pain in labor, *Wehen*, can't be traced farther back than the Middle Ages, and the word *Wehmutter* can't be found before 1540.[16]

"Also, in medieval times the Church has a service for new mothers called the 'Purification of Women,' patterned after Mary's having brought the baby Jesus to the temple for her purification. In this ceremony, one of two beautiful Psalms was read to the new mother—either Psalm 121 or Psalm 128.

"After the English Church broke with Rome, this service was included in The Book of Common Prayer[17] and has been commonly called the 'Churching of Women.' The prayer book was written during the rule of Edward VI, in 1549, and revised in 1552. In these two versions of the prayer book Psalm 128 was left out, but Psalm 121 was still used.

"But *a century later* pain in childbirth was so widely believed to be inevitable that Psalm 116 was used instead. Although this is a prayer of thanksgiving after being delivered from suffering, it has nothing to do with the birth of a child."

Pastor Dirkson opened a copy of the prayer book and explained, "From 1662 on, with few changes since, when a woman brought a baby to church after its birth this service was read to her:

> Forasmuch as it hath pleased Almighty God of His Goodness to give you safe deliverance, and hath preserved you in the great danger of childbirth; you shall therefore give hearty thanks unto God and say. . . .

> [from Psalm 116] The snares of death compassed me round and the pains of hell gat hold upon me. I found trouble and heaviness, and I called upon the name of the Lord. . . . I was in misery and he helped me. . . . Thou has delivered my soul from death.

"After the woman had repeated this passage, the following prayer was read to her:

> Oh, Almighty God, we give Thee humble thanks for that Thou hast vouchsafed to deliver this woman, Thy servant, from the great pain and peril of childbirth."

Pastor Dirkson closed the book, took off his glasses, laid them on his desk, and leaned back in his chair. "As a matter of fact," he said, "childbirth *was* a time of great pain and peril when this was written, and theologians assumed that this was true of childbirth anywhere in the world in all ages. Were there any reasons why pain might be more common at this time than in preceding centuries?"

"Well," John mused, "hard-working peasant people give birth more easily, as a rule, than the less active city people. And people left the farms in large numbers during this time to live in the cities."

"That was surely one factor. And events like the Black Death, which wiped out a third of Europe's population in the fifteenth century, the diseases and filth prevalent in the cities, all made childbirth a hazardous affair.

"But the fact that pain existed doesn't explain why it became a part of Church doctrine. This was a period of many changes in the Church—a period of reaction to the excesses of the Roman Church, which included, in the Calvinistic and Puritan movements, a rejection of anything pleasant to the senses, whether artistry, or music, or pageantry, or physical pleasures. So, although the clergy now married, a taint still remained on the functions of a *married* woman—a taint that could only be expiated by the sufferings of childbirth. Only the prostitute or mistress—never the godly wife!—ever enjoyed intercourse in such a society. Childbirth, since it involved a woman's sexual organs, shared an association with the clandestine nature of intercourse, so that the idea that childbirth was a physical experience that a woman might even *enjoy* would have been unthinkable in such a society.

"One time a young bride timidly approached her famous preacher husband and informed him that she was expecting a child. With fire in his eye, he told her never to mention such a subject to him again. And she never did, although she bore him several children."

"It's only in recent decades, isn't it," John mused, "that we've come to realize that sex in marriage is normal and wholesome, and something to be enjoyed by both husband and wife."

"Yes, John. But remember that not all Christians have shared such unwholesome attitudes in any period of Church history. But the damage of such attitudes was widespread. Today, we do have more reasonable attitudes toward sex, and toward an expectant mother, too, and I think this is one reason our society is finally beginning to move toward a more wholesome attitude about the birth process as well.

"The really sad thing to me is that although the Church has abandoned other false teachings such as flagellism, the burning of heretics, searching out witches, and the evils of marriage, it has been slower than the rest of our culture in accepting childbirth as normal. This false teaching of God's curse of pain on all mothers has been growing stronger, not weaker. We see this in the fact that where the King James translates words referring to childbirth as 'sorrow,' more recently—that is, within the last fifty years and less—translators have been changing these same words to read as 'pangs, anguish, writhing,' and even 'agony'! Can you think of any reason for this?"

"I've heard of the terrible death rate of the nineteenth century due to puerperal fever," John replied, "when up to a third of the mothers died from childbirth in some years."

"Yes. You see, along with this terrible death rate, a great fear of *dying* in childbirth developed. This great fear caused a woman to become so tense during labor that she resisted the normal progress of the birth and created agonizing experiences of suffering for herself. In this way, a vicious cycle was maintained. Probably no period in the history of the world has seen so much suffering connected with childbirth as the last century. This suffering led medical men to search for ways to relieve it, and anesthesia was discovered. But, you see, since the time its use began, until Dr. Dick-Read began his research over fifty years ago, few in our culture had even bothered to look for *normal* causes for pain in the normal physiological function of the birth of a child, because of the Church's teaching that the mother's pain was due to the 'curse of Eve,' in other words, due to the vindictiveness of God!

"Dr. Dick-Read couldn't accept this philosophy. His personal belief that God was a God of love gave him the incentive to begin, and to continue, his search for the real causes of childbirth pain. I'll give you a sample of what he says about his approach in his book, *Childbirth Without Fear*." The pastor picked up his reading glasses with one accustomed hand as he selected a book from those ranged across the entire back edge of his massive desk. "Here's the passage I wanted," he said. "Listen to this:

> My close association with the birth of a child has led me to believe there is a limitation to science, and the extending boundaries of human knowledge have only reached the foothills of the towering mountains of Omniscience. This philosophy of childbirth is written, therefore, in terms of a belief in God. . . ."[18]

"We human beings are surely ignorant, aren't we?" John commented wryly. "The Bible revealed God as a wonderful Creator and a God of love all the time—but we haven't believed it in relation to a birth. Thanks so much, pastor, for all the time you've given to help us learn the truth."

Notes

1. Rabbi Immanuel Jakobovits, *Jewish Medical Ethics, A Comparative and Historical Study of the Jewish Religious Attitude to Medicine and Its Practice* (New York: Philosophical Library, 1959), pp. 103, 104.
2. E. S. Cowles, *Religion and Medicine in the Church* (New York: Macmillan, 1925), p. 18.
3. C. Capellmann, *Pastoral-Medizin* (1878), quoted in Jakobovits, *Jewish Medical Ethics*, pp. 103, 104.
4. Jakobovits, *Jewish Medical Ethics.*
5. Clement of Alexandria, "The Instructor," Book I, Chap. VI, in *The Ante-Nicene Fathers* (Grand Rapids: Eerdmans, 1951), Vol. II, pp. 419 ff.
6. *Ibid.*
7. Clement of Rome, "The Clementine Homilies," Book XIX, Chap. XX, in *The Ante-Nicene Fathers*, Vol. VIII, pp. 173 ff.
8. Tertullian, "On the Apparel of Woman," Book I, Chap. I, in *The Ante-Nicene Fathers*, Vol. IV, p. 14.
9. Tertullian, *To His Wife*, Book I, Chap. V, and *On Exhortation to Chastity*, Chap. IX, p. 436.
10. Cyprian, "The Treatise of Cyprian," Treatise II, in *The Ante-Nicene Fathers*, Vol. V, p. 436.
11. *Ibid.*
12. *Ibid.*, Treatise IX.

13. F. W. Farrar, *Lives of the Fathers* (Edinburgh: Black, 1889), Vol. II, pp. 302, 303.
14. The Talmud (London: Soncino Press, 1936), Bereshith 17.
15. Maurice Harris, *Translations from the Talmud, Midrashim, and Kabbala* (New York: Dunne, 1901), p. 141.
16. Herr Ernst Burkhardt, who translated Dr. Dick-Read's *Childbirth Without Fear* into German, and Dr. Rudolf Hellmann, of Hamburg, in his paper *"Schmerz oder Erlebnis der Entbindung,"* January 1959, quoted in Dick-Read, *Childbirth Without Fear*, 3rd rev. ed., pp. 98, 99.
17. The Book of Common Prayer, used in the Church of England and in the Protestant Episcopal churches of the United States.
18. Grantly Dick-Read, M.D., *Childbirth Without Fear*, 4th Rev. ed. (New York: Harper & Row, 1972), p. 36.

Chapter 12

God Is My Rock

*He that dwelleth in the secret place of the most
High shall abide under the shadow of the Almighty.
I will say of the Lord, He is my refuge and my
fortress: my God; in him will I trust. Ps. 91:1, 2.*

Spring slipped softly into the countryside, touching the trees and
shrubs with her fairy's wand until they were masses of pink and
white blossoms, framed in the dainty green of new leaves. No crash-
ing storms announced her arrival—no sudden transformation from
a barren brown and white landscape to one covered with a mantle
of green. All winter long the many evergreen trees retained their
color. All winter long the lawns were green under the gentle rains.

Nowhere is spring more beautiful. One's gaze is arrested by the
stunning rose, lavender, and pink-shaded rhododendrons, each
flower so large that two hands cupped together could not contain
all its fragrant petals. Masses of roses, azaleas, and daffodils fill the
yards with the softest of pastels. Because spring tiptoes in with
utmost delicacy here, she can paint landscapes of the most fragile
beauty. A sudden transformation to such loveliness from barren
soil would be almost too much for the senses to bear.

Mary had always loved the spring, and now, this year, each
opening blossom, each little bud expanded almost to the bursting
point with new life within, reminded her of her own budding fruit.
Never before had she felt such a kinship with all nature. Never

before had she been so keenly aware of God's constant presence. She felt a peace and serenity in the knowledge of His nearness that was deeper and more meaningful than she had ever experienced before. Now that the "fruit of her womb" was almost ripe, her faith in the God who had caused it to grow there was complete.

John noticed this new serenity in Mary. He thought, as he observed his wife day after day, that perhaps many women had longed to look forward to giving birth as a natural, beautiful experience given by a loving Creator, but had hesitated to follow the leading of their hearts because they thought that this was contrary to the teaching of the Bible. He felt profoundly grateful to their pastor for his counsel in this matter.

Mary's pen, never far away, was frequently at hand now, as she tried, day after day, to express in words the beauty that filled the world around her.

One day she and John had driven out into the country and had seen frisky baby lambs gamboling on the soft grass of farm after farm. How they had laughed at one wee fellow, trying to enjoy a snack from his mother. His short legs could not keep pace with hers when he tried to reach his dinner. Skipping quickly up in front of her, he placed himself across her path and leaned against her with all his might so she would stand still. But as soon as he stopped leaning against her forelegs and ran back for his drink, she ambled on again, and he had to go without his meal.

"Apparently his mother doesn't believe in demand feeding!" John had chuckled.

The late March day had been perfect—with billowing white clouds gliding leisurely across an azure sky. Mary had tried to jot down some of her impressions of the scenery when they arrived home, but somehow, along with her inner peace and serenity, there was a restless stirring of anticipation, matched by the restless limbs of her growing baby, and she could not bring herself to concentrate on words.

One early April day as she sat on the couch watching the soothing touch of a spring rain on the beauty outside her window, she thought of Helen Keller, blind, deaf, and dumb, and she began a poem again—

You say she's blind?—
>   She who walks a country lane
>   And lifts her face to greet the rain,
> Or wanders through a garden fair
>   Inhaling all the fragrance there?

You say she's deaf?—
>   Who, standing near the ocean's roar
>   Can feel its pounding from the shore,
> Or hear . . .

But Mary could not finish it. Her expectancy had infused her with this strange paradox of feelings—restlessness, at the very time she was experiencing such peace and trust in God! This time, as she put down her pen and paper, she knew she would not try to write again until her baby was in her arms. Hearing the click of the mailbox, Mary roused herself from her reverie.

Shifting her weight a little in order to work herself up off the couch, she finally got to her feet and walked out into the hall. Returning to the room with a letter from Aunt Em in her hand, she felt a strange, uneasy premonition. She hesitated for a moment, then opened the letter and read it.

                                      Tues., April 2

Dear John and Mary,

  I am sitting by the bedside of my dear George,
as he comes to the end of his struggle for
life. He is very weak, and may leave us at any
moment. A nurse friend is here with me, and
has been such a help.

  A week ago yesterday George suffered a cerebral
spasm, and has been losing ground very constantly. We think he has not suffered, and for
this we thank God sincerely. . . .

Mary's eyes filled with tears as she read, and she could barely see to finish Aunt Em's letter.

Wed., April 3

Now I am alone. George passed quietly away in his sleep last night as we watched over him. . . . As the world judges, he has not been successful, but our intimate and family life has been unsurpassed in happiness and love. I have so many wonderful memories, and pray God for the courage to go on alone now. I know that my loved one is with his God, and that he will know "neither pain, nor sickness, nor sorrow," any more. I am determined not to weep selfish tears for my own loss, but only to rejoice for his happiness.

Lovingly,

Aunt Emma

P.S. Mary, last night George motioned toward his top dresser drawer. I followed where he pointed. Opening the drawer, I saw a slip of paper lying on some old notebooks. I brought it over to him, and, guessing what he wanted, asked, "Is this for Mary?" He nodded, pleased that I had understood, and closed his eyes, exhausted. He never opened them again.

The slip of paper had fallen to the floor unnoticed. Mary left it where it fell and hurried to the phone to call John. He came home as quickly as he could make arrangements, to find his wife in tears, Aunt Em's letter still in her hand. Guessing the contents before he opened it, he read the letter and then attempted to comfort Mary.

"You needn't worry about Aunt Em, honey," he assured her.

"She has such deep faith in God. He'll give her strength to carry on alone."

"I know, John," Mary sobbed in his arms, "but—it seemed that I was just getting to know Uncle George. He was the dearest old man! Isn't it odd that it should seem to me as if I'd known him all my life?"

"No, it's not odd," John said thoughtfully. "The more I think about it, the more I realize that you and Uncle George are kindred spirits. You're alike in many ways. Probably that's why you felt so drawn to him from the very first. By the way, where is this slip of paper Aunt Em mentions?" He looked around the room.

"Why, I don't know," Mary said, wiping her eyes. "I must have dropped it."

"Here it is." John picked it up off the floor and opened it. "It's a poem for you, Mary. Uncle George must have wanted you to have it."

Mary looked over John's arm and saw that Aunt Emma had written a note of explanation at the top of the page. "George's poem was inspired by the sight of an enormous white rock, sculptured by the ocean's waves into the shape of a great throne."

"He must have written that years ago," John exclaimed. "I remember one summer when they took me with them to the coast. Uncle George was constantly reminding me to notice this or notice that, how beautiful it was. I'll read this to you, honey." He smoothed out the creases against his knee, and read,

> The Psalmist saw a throne like this,
>   And cried in reverential bliss—
> O God, of great eternal power,
>   Thou art my Rock, and my High Tower!
>
> A fortress Thou, O God, above;
>   Thee will I trust, and Thee I'll love.
> On Thee I'll call, and Thee I'll praise,
>   To Thee my hands with reverence raise.
> When in distress I'll cry to Thee,
>   For Thou, O God, wilt succor me.

Upon my knees I'll worship Thee
Sing forth Thy praise continually.
O God, of great and mighty power—
Thou are my Rock, and my High Tower!

Mary's tears had dried on her cheeks as she listened. "Uncle George is in the shadow of that Rock now, isn't he?—more completely than at any time he was living here."

"Yes," said John. "It's a wonderful thing to be a Christian, isn't it, Mary? To know that when this life ends, our fullest life is just beginning."

That evening, as Mary and John took their daily walk, Uncle George and Aunt Emma were still very much in their thoughts. John patiently slowed his steps to Mary's and walked beside his very pregnant wife with a sense of protectiveness and pride. They stopped often along the quiet streets to look up through the lacy network of new leaves on old trees, silhouetted against the sky, with the moon, dimmed by passing clouds, shining softly through. All around them was evidence of the constant love and mercy of God. They realized anew that the beauty of this life, which comes from God, is but a shadow of the beauty of the life to come, where is needed "no candle, neither light of the sun; for the Lord God giveth them light. . . ." And they realized again that after night, comes morning; and after winter, spring; and after death, the Resurrection.

Chapter 13

In Quietness and in Confidence

*Thou wilt keep him in perfect peace, whose mind
is stayed on Thee, because he trusteth in Thee.* Isa.
26:3.

Easter had come and gone. Each passing day seemed longer to
Mary than the one before. She tried to forget the calendar and
keep busy, but her eager anticipation of the arrival of her baby
occupied her thoughts and left little room for enthusiasm over any
other project.

Space was at a premium in their little bedroom, with the bassinet
and baby's dresser fitted into the only empty corners of the room.
The dresser drawers were bulging with the many gifts Mary's
friends had given her at a shower, and she had gone over each item
many times, fingering the woven softness of sacques and booties,
or the silken delicacy of bonnets and blankets.

Thursday morning as Mary washed the few breakfast dishes,
she glanced frequently out the window at the bright April landscape, hoping that April might not slip over into May before her
baby had arrived. She was glad that she and John had had a chance
to visit the maternity section of the hospital and see a film on the
birth of a baby. John had also gone with her on her last visit to the
doctor, although he hadn't gone with her every time. On impulse,
Mary dried her hands suddenly, went into the bedroom and returned
with the instructions the doctor had given her to study a couple of
months before.

These reminded her to report at once any persistent headache, swelling, puffiness, or sudden weight gain, and any bleeding or premature breaking of the waters (fluid from the sac in which the baby had been growing). They told her of the three signs of labor she was to watch for and report to him:

1. A pinkish discharge from the vagina, known as "the show." This is the "plug" that has kept the cervix closed in pregnancy.
2. Leaking of fluid from the sac, which may rupture suddenly with a rush of fluid, or from which the water may leak slowly.
3. The beginning of contractions. These are felt as *a slight tightening and pressure in the lower abdomen just above the pelvic bone.* A slight pressure may also be felt on the lower back, making one sit up a bit straighter.

If this tightening low in the abdomen is felt occurring at intervals of ten to fifteen or twenty minutes, it is time to call the doctor. Being relaxed and confident, having prepared for a natural birth, *do not think that you are not really in labor because the contractions are not painful,* or you may end up having your husband help you deliver your baby unexpectedly at home!

Dr. Gordon had told them that when he first began training his patients for natural childbirth, he found many of them coming to the hospital far advanced in labor, so that he really had to rush to deliver their babies in time. Neither he nor the mothers had realized that they were so near delivery, because they had had no discomfort. He told Mary *not* to go to bed to relax while still at home when her labor began, but to stay up. The slight tension which this involved would make her more aware of contractions, so that she would know when to go to the hospital. If she learned the signs of labor well, she needn't worry about knowing when to go. Occasionally even the best laid plans go awry, however, so he asked Mary to memorize the rules to follow in case of emergency birth.

She held the sheet in her hand, but looked out the kitchen window absently as she went over the instructions from memory:

1. Remain quiet and confident. Millions of women before you have borne their babies in this natural manner.

2. Brace yourself in a semisitting position on a padded surface (such as a folded blanket, covered by newspapers or a clean sheet), your back supported by large pillows or by a wall. *Do not lie down on your back!*

3. Draw up your knees, grasp them with your hands, take a deep breath, and bear down gently with each contraction. (These instructions assume that the first stage of labor and the transition period have passed and that the baby has descended into the birth canal, ready to be born.)

4. As you feel the baby's head about to be born, *stop pushing*, and pant with short breaths in the upper chest, so the baby will be born slowly by uterine contraction alone.

5. Support baby's head with your hand as it begins to emerge, holding it *up* and toward you over the pubic bone so you will not tear. Support his body also as it follows. Baby will rotate as he is born until he is facing you.

6. Break the bag of waters and remove baby immediately if he is born in it, so he will not drown as he draws his first breath. Lay baby over your abdomen, his head lower than his body, and clear his air passages so he can breathe, by wiping away any mucus.

7. If baby doesn't breathe at once (he nearly always does, after a spontaneous birth), keep his head low and spank his heels. If this doesn't work, do mouth-to-mouth breathing, through a clean handkerchief, if available. Cover both his mouth and nose with your mouth and blow gently into his lungs rhythmically for as long as necessary.

8. Wrap baby warmly in whatever is handy, put him to the breast at once if the cord is long enough (*never pull on it!*), and cough gently with each contraction to aid in expelling the afterbirth. Be patient—this may take five minutes to an hour.

9. Wrap up the afterbirth with the baby (he won't mind!) without tying or cutting the cord, until scissors and string can be sterilized for doing so, or until medical help is available.

10. Keep the uterus round and hard to prevent bleeding by massaging it gently from time to time. Let baby nurse frequently, and you may get up and walk around as soon and as frequently as you wish.

Mary was satisfied that she knew the rules well without looking at them; she put the papers away, knowing she was prepared for any contingency. After finishing the few dishes she had left, she picked up a baby jacket she was making, sat down in a comfortable chair, and as she knit continued to think back over the things the doctor had explained on the last office visit.

Mary was to be propped up in a semisitting position for the birth, he had told her and John, because women have instinctively used variations of this position for centuries. They have apparently found it the most comfortable and the one in which they can push to best advantage. The doctor explained that it takes much less energy to push an object *down* than it does to push it straight out parallel to the ground. Even animals wisely use the aid of gravity in delivering their young.

"You won't be tied down in any way during the birth, Mary," he assured her. "Dr. Dick-Read says that he has *never* tied down a pair of arms and legs![1] The stirrups will be kept low so that you can bend your head forward and draw your knees up toward your chest while bearing down. Your arms will be free so that, when pushing, you can bend your elbows slightly outward and grasp the supports with your hands, or hold your husband's arm or hands for support, whichever you wish. Just remember not to touch the sterile area. You'll be able to rest by moving your legs as is necessary for your comfort and by relaxing against the back rest between contractions."

Dr. Gordon said he hoped to be able to deliver Mary's baby without cutting her perineum. "A friend of mine who has attended the delivery of from six hundred to seven hundred babies in Africa told me," he said, "that she had never seen a third-degree laceration, and that fewer than ten times had she felt it necessary to perform an episiotomy. Her record is better than mine," he admitted to them, smiling, "but her success has given me incentive to learn how to control the actual birth better, so that the mother will be spared the unnatural discomfort of the stitches afterward. If I do feel it necessary to make an incision, Mary, you won't feel it. One doctor has told his patients that he'll even refund their fees if they can tell when he cuts them. They can't! This is because the perineum is insensitive during the birth, although feeling returns to it almost immediately afterward."

"What about hypnosis, Dr. Gordon?" John asked. "Many of our

friends, when they hear that Mary's to have a natural birth, shrug their shoulders and say, 'Oh, that's only hypnotism.' "

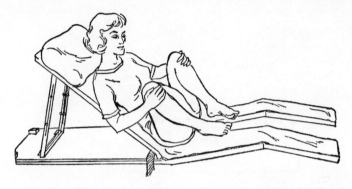

Fig. 8. Natural childbirth patient bearing down in raised position. In the absence of something to push her feet against, she may grip her knees as shown, pulling them widely apart as she bears down.

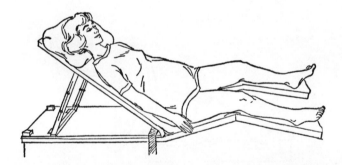

Fig. 9. Natural childbirth patient resting in raised position. It is important to have the knees supported slightly above the level of the hips in order to relax the legs completely. This is the "reclining-chair" position for relaxation during pregnancy also.

Dr. Gordon explained that only people ignorant of the phenomena of either hypnosis or natural childbirth, or both, confuse the two. "One obstetrician, who is also a trained medical hypnotist (using hypnotism for nervous personality disorders), told me that using hypnosis for obstetrics rather than preparing for a natural birth, was like using a cannon to shoot a sparrow when a simple BB gun would do the job!"[2]

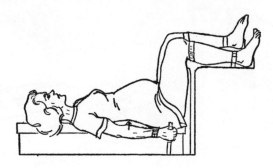

Fig. 10. Wrong position for bearing down. Notice how the mother arches her back in order to push. This position for bearing down is not only exhausting and ineffective but causes severe backache the next day.

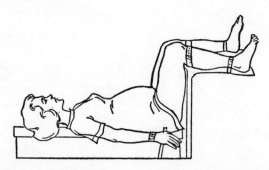

Fig. 11. Obstetric patient in wrong position on delivery table attempting to rest between contractions. Notice that she is completely unable to change position.

Then Dr. Gordon went on to explain that his main objection to people's confusing natural childbirth with autosuggestion, or with hypnotism, was that this was an inconsistent philosophy for a Christian.

"Is God responsible for pain in the normal physiological function of birth?" he asked them. "We know the Bible doesn't teach this. But how then can a Christian be unwilling to believe that pain in childbirth can be prevented by following commonsense preparation during pregnancy?

"A real drawback to using hypnosis," he told them earnestly, "is that, like anesthetics or local injections, it robs the mother of the true sensations of feeling her child born. We could learn from some of the primitive races in this, if we only would. In these cultures, women are helped by other women, who know from experience what it feels like to give birth to a child and who understand what is in a woman's mind during that time.

"In our mechanically minded American society, we doctors have tended to look with microscopic concern at all the physical details of a birth, but we've only recently been learning what the midwife has known all along—that childbirth is a great deal more than just a physical event. It's an experience of tremendous emotional and sexual significance in a woman's life. Do you remember what I told you about this in our discussion before your marriage?"

Both John and Mary replied that they did.

"This physical and emotional pleasure," the doctor said, "like the pleasant stimulation a mother receives in suckling her child later, is as pure and right in God's sight as the physical pleasure she derives from stroking the tiny limbs of her baby with her fingers, or feeling the soft whisper of his breath against her cheek. It is our Creator who has made a mother so."

Mary glanced at the clock. Only ten o'clock—the morning was passing slowly. She decided to walk over to Carolyn's for a few minutes, and ask her about a few more things still on her mind. She put her knitting away and slipped into a jacket.

The air was mild and fragrant. Mary walked slowly, enjoying every minute of it. The words of a little poem that John had found and brought to her one day came to her mind, and she held her head a little higher, confident and happy, as the charming words repeated themselves in her mind:

> She carries life in her body
> as a girl in a dry country carries

a pitcher of water cupped in her hands
delighting
the thirsty eyes of the dwellers
in those parched lands.

She is as quiet and as certain
as Earth in reluctant spring,
which waits for a night of warm showers
dissolving
the last delay of winter
and dazzling the dawn with flowers.[3]

"Come on out to the backyard, Mary," Carolyn greeted her as she stood at the door. "Greg's in his playpen, and Julie and Paul are digging in the sand." She led Mary through the house and on out to the backyard, where they could watch the children playing. Carolyn thoughtfully brought out a straight-backed chair for Mary, before jackknifing herself into one of the garden chairs.

"You look good, Mary," she told her. "Is everything okay?"

"Sure is," Mary smiled, "except that I'm getting impatient. And I can't sleep on my back any more—the baby's too heavy on my spine."

"Don't you use the side position you've learned for relaxing?" Carolyn asked. "That's what I did. It was the only way I could sleep without having to shift positions every little while and keep Ralph awake."

"The only trouble with that," Mary confided, "is that when I'm sprawled out with my knee up on an extra pillow in the bed, there's hardly room for John! He's pushed over into one narrow strip of bed. I've told him I wouldn't mind if he'd sleep on the couch, but he says he doesn't mind being crowded."

"Of course *you* didn't offer to sleep on the couch, did you?" Carolyn teased her.

"No, it's too narrow," Mary laughed. "I'd have to lie on my back, and that's not comfortable." She hesitated a moment, and then said, "I'd like to ask you about a couple more things, Carolyn."

"Okay, shoot," Carolyn said agreeably.

Mary sat up a bit straighter as the jab of a little foot reminded her that things were getting pretty crowded in the warm nest of her baby. "What do the nurses mean when they talk about 'prepping'?" she asked.

"Well, some doctors have a nurse prep the patient by shaving off the pubic hair and giving an enema. But Dr. Gordon doesn't usually order this for his patients. From time to time the nurses will examine you to see how far the cervix has opened. They're not permitted to make a vaginal examination, as they might cause an infection, so they do this by inserting a finger into the rectum, and feeling the size of the cervical opening through its wall."

"I've heard those rectal exams are really awful," Mary said, looking worried.

"They're not awful unless you tighten up and resist them because of embarrassment. But there's really no need to be embarrassed— the nurses do this so often they don't think any more about it than I do about changing my babies. Their minds are more likely to be on what they ought to fix for supper, or what they should wear to go out that evening. Anyway, Dr. Gordon has taught the nurses to tell how far along the mother is by observing her actions, so they make internal examinations much less frequently."

"Then I'll just relax and let them do whatever they want with me!"

"That's the spirit, Mary. You can put up with little annoyances like these good-naturedly. Excuse me a minute!"

Carolyn jumped up to pick Julie off the fence. She scolded her daughter, set her back in the sandbox, and put the baby's toys back in his playpen before returning to her chair. Baby Greg solemnly began dropping his toys outside his playpen again, one by one, as soon as her back was turned.

Carolyn curled up in her chair, casting a weather eye at her young daughter again. "Julie!" she warned. Julie obediently climbed back into the sandbox with Paul, deciding to wait for a more opportune moment, when her mother wasn't watching, to climb back up the fence.

"Let's see. Where were we?" Carolyn pondered. "Oh, yes. I

wanted to tell you that there are two things about a natural birth which hurt some. The first is the spraying of the antiseptic solution on the pubic area after you're taken into the delivery room. That really stings! I wish some of our brilliant scientists would do some research on an antiseptic without a sting!"

Mary laughed appreciatively. "What's the other thing?"

"The other is the injection of the Novocain needle if any stitches are needed afterward. The perineum has no sensation during the birth but is very sensitive shortly afterward, as its circulation is re-established."

"What if you'd had a breech baby? Would Dr. Gordon still have let you have a natural birth?"

"Oh, yes. He explained to me that the only difference is that a breech birth takes longer, since the baby's soft bottom doesn't dilate either the cervix or the perineum as well as his hard head. Of course, a longer labor is no more uncomfortable if you know how to relax. There's often more backache with a breech, though, especially during transition, so someone needs to massage the mother's back during more of her labor. You can trust Dr. Gordon, Mary, to do his best to help you have the kind of experience you want. He won't spoil it for you unless he has a good reason."

"Carolyn, you've been such a help to me all along. I don't know how to thank you," Mary said earnestly, as she rose to leave.

"My best thanks would be for you to have a happy experience like mine," Carolyn smiled, as she walked with her around the house. She waved good-bye as Mary went down the walk, before returning to her own little ones in the backyard.

Notes

1. Grantly Dick-Read, M.D., *Childbirth Without Fear*, 4th rev. ed. (New York: Harper & Row, 1972), p. 289.
2. Reported in *Child-Family Digest*, September-October 1960.
3. Written by Alexander Scott, printed in *A Book of Scotland*, ed. G. F. Maine (London: Collins, 1950), pp. 339, 340. Reprinted by permission.

Chapter 14

The Gift of God

Every good gift and every perfect gift is from above, and cometh down from the Father of lights, with whom is no variableness, neither shadow of turning. James 1:17.

Once again Mary shifted in her sleep. The first streaks of dawn were appearing across the morning sky. She glanced at her watch—five o'clock, it said. She lay back, wondering why she felt restless. She placed her hand on her abdomen, feeling for a contraction, but there was nothing. Finally she drifted back to sleep.

"Are you all right, Mary?" John asked her at the breakfast table later. "You seemed restless last night." He looked at her anxiously, but she seemed relaxed and cheerful.

"I'm fine," she assured him, sitting up a little straighter in her chair as she felt a fleeting pressure on her lower back.

"You're sure you don't want me to stay home today?"

"Oh, no, John."

"Be sure to call me if your labor starts, honey. The principal said he'd arrange for my classes if I had to leave during the school day."

"I will. Please, don't fret so about me."

"Promise?"

"I promise. I'll call you right away."

John kissed her good-bye and reluctantly started off to his classes. Mary picked up some of the breakfast dishes and carried them to the sink. Instinctively she stopped in the middle of the room, as she felt her lower abdomen tighten a bit. She glanced at the clock. Eight-twenty, it said. The feeling passed, and she went on with her work.

Eight-thirty. She had glanced at the clock again. Wouldn't it be exciting if my baby was to be born today? she thought dreamily, picturing him already cradled in the curve of her arm, or nestled against her shoulder. Her heart skipped a beat in sudden elation. She wondered if she should call the doctor—although she was sure these little twinges couldn't be labor!

Eight-forty. This time Mary went to the phone. Dr. Gordon advised her to come right over to the hospital.

Mary called John, who had just arrived at school. He was home again within a few minutes. He picked up her overnight case, they climbed into the car, and he began driving madly toward the hospital.

"Please don't drive so fast!" Mary gasped, stiffening because of a very uncomfortable contraction. She gripped the arm rest of the car tensely, to keep from being jarred with every rise in the pavement. John slowed down and drove more carefully. In his mind he had pictured the baby as arriving at any minute, and he was anxious to get to the hospital in time.

As they reached the hospital approach, another contraction began, unmistakable this time, and Mary again braced herself stiffly against it. As soon as it had passed, they entered the hospital and walked up to the receiving desk.

They gave their names at the desk, and a nurse brought a wheelchair for Mary. She disdained it, however, preferring to walk.

Miss Elleson greeted them at the door of the labor ward and ushered them into a room. After seeing where Mary was to be, John returned to the receiving desk to complete their registration. Mary undressed quickly, slipped into a hospital gown, and Miss Elleson, cheerful and efficient, soon had her comfortable. She left Mary to get her an extra pillow, assuring her that the doctor would be in shortly.

Just as Miss Elleson went out the door, Mary was very startled by the sac rupturing suddenly, and the clean bedding was flooded with water. Although she had known this would happen, it had surprised her by its suddenness, and she was also dismayed at having drenched the bedclothes.

"I'm so terribly sorry!" she apologized to Miss Elleson, as the latter returned with a pillow.

"Don't give it a thought, Mrs. Thomas," Miss Elleson assured her. "This happens to everybody, and we don't mind a bit." She changed the bedding quickly and soon had Mary comfortable again.

"It's more restful to shift positions occasionally," she advised Mary, "but keep your joints—like knees and elbows—flexed a little, as this helps you to relax. And be sure to keep your bladder and bowels empty, so you can keep the birth outlet as loosely relaxed as possible. Call me for this as often as you need to. That's what I'm here for." She gave Mary a reassuring smile. "Would you like to turn over and slip the extra pillow under your knee now?"

"I'm comfortable just now, thank you," Mary said politely. After Miss Elleson had gone out, Mary studied the room as she waited for John and the doctor to come. The walls were a soft pastel, and there were *pictures*! Mary had never thought there would be pictures hanging in a labor room. She closed her eyes, took two or three deep breaths, and allowed herself to go limp as a contraction came on. When it had passed, she studied the pictures contentedly. One was the lovely "Madonna of the Streets," the other a chubby little boy asleep on his tummy, his knees tucked under him, his little round bottom making a hump under his blankets.

Mary turned her gaze toward the windows and discovered that they were framed with flowered material and that she could see the green tips of the trees in the courtyard below. The harmonious atmosphere of the room gave her a feeling of peace and quiet anticipation.

Miss Elleson ushered John into the room to be with Mary. There was a lounge chair for him in the corner, with a magazine rack, but he chose a straight-back chair instead, and drew it up close beside the bed.

"Everything okay?" he asked Mary.

"Yes, honey. Isn't this a pretty room? By the way," she said, turning toward the nurse, "this is Miss Elleson, John. She's been so nice to me. This is my husband, Miss Elleson."

"I assumed that!" the nurse replied, a mischievous twinkle in her eye. A moment later she left them alone.

"John, d'you know what?" Mary mused thoughtfully. "I wasn't the least bit relaxed on the way to the hospital, was I?"

"You sure weren't! You were hanging on for dear life!"

"No wonder those contractions were so uncomfortable!" she said soberly. "I was holding on so I wouldn't be jarred—but it made my contractions hurt. I'm sure glad I've learned how to relax. I can see how *awful* labor could be if you started out all tensed up like that and didn't know how to relax!" Mary placed her hand absently over her abdomen, and was surprised to find it hard as a rock beneath her touch.

"Why," she exclaimed in surprise, "I must be having a contraction right now, and I didn't even know it!"

"You've had a little time to quiet down," John smiled at her. He put his face down close to her cheek, and said softly by her ear as he stroked her hair lovingly, "Remember, honey, not to be afraid to trust the God Who made you! Just sink down into His arms, and everything will be all right."

Mary nodded peacefully. A moment later Dr. Gordon entered the room. "Miss Elleson tells me your cervix is beginning to dilate, Mary, so we're on our way all right." He bent over her to check the baby's position and heartbeat. "Seems fine," he commented.

"This is such a nice room, Dr. Gordon," Mary told him. "I feel as if I were in a guest room—not in a hospital!"

Dr. Gordon smiled appreciatively. "We want the mothers to feel that they're guests. They're certainly not invalids!" He sat down on the edge of the bed and visited a few minutes. His calm conversation and explanations were reassuring to both Mary and John. Now whenever Mary became conscious of a contraction beginning, she took a few slow, relaxed breaths and let her whole body sag. Between them she chatted happily. The doctor stayed long enough to observe Mary unobtrusively during her contractions. He was pleased to note that she was relaxing properly, and complimented her.

"Turn over onto your left side soon now, Mary, and see if you can relax enough to doze a while. The less you think about your uterus now, the more quickly it'll open the door for you. After a while," he explained, "you'll notice that the contractions will become much longer and closer together for a few minutes, and you'll feel more pressure on your lower spine. This is the transition period, during which you'll begin to feel the need to change from relaxing to pushing during the contractions.

"I want you to watch for this, too, John," he said, turning to him. "You can help Mary tell when it's near by timing the length of her contractions after a while, and by noticing when it gets harder for her to relax. If her back bothers her, you can help by pressing firmly with the heel of your hand where she shows you and rotating your hand gently in a semicircular motion. Please call one of the nurses right away if you see these things before they do, and have them call me."

Turning to Mary, he said, "I have to go over to the office this morning, but I'll be prepared to leave at any time. I try to be with my patients from the transition period on through the birth, and I won't come flying in the last minute just before your baby's born— unless you pull a fast one on me. Occasionally a patient likes to make a liar out of me!" he admitted wryly, as he went out the door.

Miss Elleson returned to the room after the doctor had gone and helped Mary turn onto her left side, adjusting the pillow under her right knee and thigh until she was comfortable. She pointed to a can of talcum powder and suggested to John that he use it for Mary if she needed her back massaged.

The minutes ticked by. Mary let herself become limper and limper until she was barely aware of the contractions at all. Finally she drifted off into a light sleep. John picked up a magazine and relaxed in the lounge chair, keeping a weather eye on his wife. Time crept by at a snail's pace for him.

Several hours passed. Miss Elleson looked in frequently but, seeing Mary dozing, went out again. Mary opened her eyes finally, feeling refreshed. "I guess I didn't sleep much last night," she admitted. John moved quickly back to her side.

Miss Elleson came in. She noticed that a flush had come into Mary's cheeks (a sign that the cervix is about three-fifths dilated), so she went out again without making an internal examination to determine the progress of the labor.

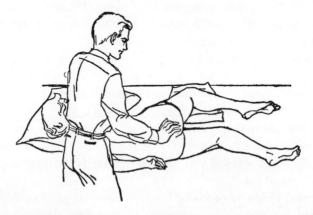

Fig. 12. Husband of natural childbirth patient rubbing her back correctly, using a semicircular motion and pressing firmly with the heel of his hand.

"You ought to go to supper," Mary said, worrying about John. "It's getting late."

"I'm staying right here!" he responded, so firmly that she didn't question it. Secretly she was relieved that he hadn't left her.

A few moments later Miss Elleson appeared again with a glass of orange juice for Mary. "Would you like a supper tray sent up for you?" she asked, turning to John, and he readily agreed.

After finishing his supper, John pulled out his watch, slipped his left hand under Mary's abdomen, and timed her contractions for a while. They were now less than five minutes apart. Mary lay quietly as a couple more hours passed. Suddenly she stiffened.

"My back! Please rub it, honey." John put down the watch, stood up and rubbed furiously, anxious to be of help, and glad that he could do something more at last.

"You're about to shove me through the bed," Mary objected, "and you don't need to—" she caught her breath "—rub my skin off!" She held her breath and waited for the long, powerful contraction to pass. "I can't relax," she complained, stiffening, as another strong contraction followed a few seconds later. John realized that she had reached the transition stage, and as soon as the contraction ended, stepped out into the hall, returning with a different nurse.

"Where's Miss Elleson?" Mary asked crossly.

"She'll be here in a minute," the new nurse said pleasantly. "She's calling Dr. Gordon. Keep your abdominal wall completely relaxed, Mrs. Thomas, and breathe in and out more deeply and quickly during the next contraction." She pressed her hand firmly on Mary's lower back and watched carefully to be sure that Mary did not begin breathing the shallow, rapid breaths that indicate tension. "Stay relaxed and breathe *deeply* now, in, out, in, out. That's it, not too fast." Mary found that following the nurse's instructions kept her relaxed and comfortable throughout the contraction.

When it ended, the nurse suggested she turn onto her back, and raised the head of the bed to the reclining-chair position. She rolled pillows into bolsters, and placed them under Mary's knees. Mary found this semisitting position far more comfortable at this stage of labor, and again let her muscles become relaxed and limp. Dr. Gordon arrived in the room just then and coached her breathing through the next contraction. Mary found that sitting up partially like this not only made it easier to relax but seemed to relieve the pressure on her back.

"This transition will be over shortly," Dr. Gordon assured her, "and then you'll feel much better. Would you like a whiff of gas?"

Mary shook her head. "I don't need it, but I'm cold," she complained, "and I c-can't stop my l-legs shaking." The nurses quickly covered her more warmly. Mary began to breathe properly again as the next contraction started, but to her surprise the contraction ended abruptly, and she cried in relief, "There! That's better!" The baby's head had slipped on through the cervix into the birth canal, and she was immediately more comfortable. Emotionally keyed up from the excitement of the transition period, she grabbed her knees and pushed down with all her might.

"No, my dear," Dr. Gordon chided her gently. "Just lie back and rest a bit. The contractions will come farther apart now. Push only when you feel one beginning, and if it hurts to push, don't push at all, but wait until it feels comfortable to do it."

Mary relaxed against the pillow behind her head on the back rest. Opening her eyes, she was surprised to find John standing just beside her left arm, dressed in hospital regalia. She had temporarily forgotten all about him.

"You sure make a handsome intern!" she teased him. He bowed deeply in mock acknowledgment of the compliment.

"Thank you, madam," he replied solemnly.

Just then Mary felt a contraction beginning. Again she gripped the supports and strained as hard as she could. She was amazed at how good it felt to bear down! But again she became aware of the doctor saying something to her. As the contraction ended, she gave him her full attention.

"When a contraction begins, Mary," he was saying, "take a cleansing in-and-out breath; then take a deep breath, hold it, and lean over and push gently, keeping the birth outlet completely slack and limp as you push. Take another breath or two during the contraction if necessary. Push firmly, but don't strain. Have you read the Bible verse that says, 'Man that is born of a woman . . . cometh forth like a flower?' "

Mary shook her head as she watched him, interested.

"Think of yourself as a flower, too," he told her. "In films that show a flower opening we see its petals unfold a bit, rest, open, rest, open, slowly, irresistibly, rhythmically, in the steady, even rhythm of all growing things. Mrs. Dick-Read says that a mother giving birth should think of herself as 'a rose unfolding.' " His quiet tone was reassuring to Mary.

As each contraction began, John slipped his right arm around Mary's shoulders and helped her lean over to push. She gripped her knees, pulled them up toward her shoulders, took a deep breath, held it, took another, held it, then let it out in a soft, moaning sigh as the contraction ended. She sank back peacefully onto the back rest, took two or three deep in-and-out breaths to replace her oxygen and cleanse her lungs, and then relaxed limply as she waited for the next contraction. She was grateful that she did not have to be moved to another room for the birth, but could stay where she was. Dr. Gordon had explained that throughout most of the world, mothers were permitted to stay in the same bed throughout labor and birth if all was going well.

"You may have a whiff of gas any time you want one," a nurse reminded her.

"Thank you, but I don't need it!" Mary replied, not too graciously. An hour passed by quietly. Like a lovely flower, Mary thought. There's one! Deep breath—push, push—rest! —Push! —Rest! —Push! —Rest!

There was no unnecessary noise. Dr. Gordon and John conversed quietly from time to time, but Mary didn't mind. She seemed oblivious to all that went on most of the time, but actually she was acutely aware of every slight sound or motion in the room. She just did not bother to respond.

She was perspiring freely now, and John tenderly wiped the perspiration from her forehead with some tissues from a box set near him, each time she sank back after bearing down. Once he leaned over and whispered to her softly, "The 'renunciation of toil,' Mary?"

She nodded happily, turning her smiling face toward him without opening her eyes. ". . . labor of love," she murmured.

Again she felt the impulse to bear down strongly, and this time as she did so she experienced a new sensation—a bulging feeling at the outlet of the birth canal. "Look here, Mary," someone was saying.

She opened her eyes and noticed that a mirror had been adjusted so that she could see the top of a little head appearing. She roused from her half-stupor and cried excitedly, "The baby! Oh! Look, John! The baby! It has black hair!" She worked with a will now, with a mounting excitement, and soon began to feel a pins and needles sensation at the outlet. "It's such a bursting feeling," she gasped, short of breath, as the contraction passed. She appeared alarmed.

"Does it hurt?" Dr. Gordon asked quietly.

"No," Mary answered thoughtfully, and then smiled. "I guess I'm just afraid it's *going* to hurt!"

"Keep the birth outlet as limp as you can," Dr. Gordon said quietly, "and the prickly feeling will be gone in a few seconds now. Don't push any more, but pant during contractions. Take little short breaths in your upper chest with your mouth open, breathing *out, out, out*."

Mary did this during the next contraction. She found it difficult to keep from pushing.

"If you push now, you may tear," Dr. Gordon explained. "In England, you know, a midwife considers it a disgrace if she lets a mother tear. She tells the mother to let her baby's head be born 'hair by hair.' "

"You're the funniest-looking English midwife I ever saw!" Mary teased him unexpectedly. Everyone laughed, including the nurses. They especially enjoyed the joke on the doctor.

As another contraction began, Mary closed her eyes and panted, an exciting tension mounting in her head till it seemed about to burst with emotion. So hard not to push—such a tight, bulging— "There! There!" she cried happily, as the baby's head slipped into the open. Disdaining the mirror, she looked down with awe at her very own baby appearing.

"John! Look! The baby!" A moment later the doctor eased the baby's shoulders through and then told Mary she could push again during the next contraction. A tingling flush of hot warmth engulfed her whole body from head to toe as she felt her baby slipping smoothly through the vagina, and a few seconds later the young Thomas had made his debut into the world.

The baby was laid on the bed at the level of the placenta, until the cord stopped pulsing.

"Isn't he *beautiful*, John!" breathed Mary delightedly. "Isn't he a *beautiful* baby!"

John studied the red, wrinkled face of his newborn son, the black hair plastered to the little head covered with its own brand of white baby cream, and laughed indulgently. He thought to himself that the baby looked more like a greased monkey! At least it was a boy! Secretly he had hoped for a boy—someone to take to ball games—go on hikes.

As soon as the cord—which was a surprisingly pretty turquoise blue, had been tied and cut, the baby, mewing like a tiny kitten, was wrapped in a prewarmed blanket and given to Mary. And Baby Thomas, so recently thrust abruptly from the warm security of his mother's body into the cold, empty world, stopped his whimpering and nestled contentedly in the warm security of his mother's loving arms.

As Mary looked down at the tiny bundle in her arms, such a wave of happiness swept over her that she could not keep the tears from streaming down her cheeks.

"Why, Mary! What's wrong?" John asked, alarmed.

"It's—nothing," Mary sobbed. It's just that—I've never been so happy!"

As John daubed uselessly at her tears with his handkerchief, he surreptitiously brushed a tear from his own eye. A hush had come over the room, as he bent tenderly over his wife and newborn son. And for one long moment all were vividly aware of another Presence that filled the room—the eternal Spirit of the living God.

Chapter 15

The "Little Bitsa Baby, in His Hand"

Can a woman forget her sucking child, that she should not have compassion on the son of her womb? Yea, they may forget, yet will I not forget thee. Isa. 49:15.

"You certainly don't look as if you'd just had a baby!" one of the new mothers exclaimed, as a radiant Mary walked into the room she was to share.

"I don't feel like it either!" Mary answered happily. "It's like a dream my baby's already here. Didn't it all go so *fast,* John?"

John smiled but didn't reply. Time had crawled along for him as he had kept patient vigil beside his sweetheart, but, then, she had been busy and less aware of the fourteen hours of time.

Miss Jones turned down the sheets of the bed and laid Mary's son beside her after she was comfortable. "Any time you're tired," she instructed Mary, "just put your baby in this drawer-bassinet, and push it through this opening in the wall into the nursery on the other side. As soon as you do, a light will go on so we know he's there, and we'll look after him while you rest. Are you sure you don't want me to put him in his bed now?"

"Oh, please, no," Mary pleaded. She was still too excited to want to rest.

"All right," the nurse said agreeably. Before she left the room she handed Mary a sheet of instructions covering both hospital regulations and how to care for herself.

After the nurse had gone, John pulled up a chair in order to see his new son better.

"Would you like to hold him, honey?" Mary asked.

"No—no thanks," John demurred hastily, fearing lest the fragile little thing fall apart in his hands.

"The nurses will show you how to hold him properly and how to dress him," one of Mary's roommates spoke up, "and how to bathe him too. This is a wonderful hospital to be in with a new baby. We have our own dining hall and lounge, so we can be up as much as we like. And our husbands can even come see us any time between ten in the morning and eighty-thirty at night, as long as they scrub their hands and put on a hospital gown before coming in, so they can hold their babies."

"Aren't there any visiting hours?" Mary asked her.

"Oh, yes, for other visitors, because the babies aren't allowed in the room while they're here. But husbands can wander in and out any time they like."

"How nice," Mary sighed happily. "But, of course, you can't get here till after school anyway, John."

"I'll run up during the lunch hour," he assured her. "Your folks'll be here tomorrow, too, during visiting hours."

"Were they excited when you told them about the baby?"

"*Were* they! Your mother sounded as if she was crying over the phone when I told her what an easy time you'd had and how happy you were. She was awfully worried about you, Mary."

"I know." Mary stroked the baby's petal-soft cheek with her finger as she said soberly, "I tried to tell Mother that God meant giving birth to be a beautiful experience, but she was afraid to believe it for me." Mary had scarcely lifted her eyes from God's sweet gift to her since he had been put beside her, but now she looked up at John, and he took courage to reach over and slip his finger into a tiny fist.

"Wow! You wouldn't think such a delicate thing could have such a grip!" he said proudly. "Boy, will he ever be able to clutch a bat!" He turned the blanket back to study the pink feet. "All eleven toes are there, all right."

"What?" Mary nearly sat upright in bed, astonished.

"I'm joking, hon. He's only got ten. By the way, your folks wanted to know what name we had decided on. I told them we'd talked about Susan, Jane, Robert, Peter, Nancy, Walter, Linda, Nelly, Tom, Kirk, Scott, Douglas, and on, and on, and on, but that you'd never been able to make up your mind!"

"At least it won't be Susan, or Jane, or Nancy!" Mary smiled. "We really ought to decide, though," she said, more soberly. "What does he look like his name should be?"

John looked at his son thoughtfully for awhile. "It ought to be a distinguished name," he observed, "something like, 'Gregory Piedmont Beadlehouser Thomas the First'?"

But Mary didn't laugh. "I like the name Gregory," she said, "only Carolyn has a Greg, too." A thoughtful look had come over her face. "John?"

"Yes?" he answered expectantly, sensing her earnestness.

"I have an idea." Mary paused, tore her loving gaze from her baby's face and looked right into her husband's eyes. "I don't know what you'll think of it, honey," she told him seriously, "but I'd like to name our baby George."

It had been an exciting day. Mary napped a bit after John left. By suppertime she felt famished and really enjoyed her meal. Janice Wells, in the bed next to hers, told her that all the hospital meals were just as delicious and such a nice change from the constant planning and cooking at home.

Janice had a new baby girl, her second child. The baby was unusually beautiful for a newborn, with pink-white skin, lovely curling lashes, and dark hair so long its silken folds brushed against her dainty neck.

Elaine Dieple was Mary's other roommate, the mother of five children now. The three of them had talked on into the evening on the universal topics of discussion in maternity wards everywhere —their labors, their babies, and the things they liked or didn't like about their doctors!

Elaine had had a natural birth, like Mary's. Janice had had a long, painful labor in spite of deep sedation, and had had a saddle block at birth. All three of them planned to nurse their babies.

Finally, Elaine and Janice turned out their lights, but Mary, still refreshed from her recent nap, left hers on for a few more minutes in order to read over the instructions the nurse had given her earlier. She was especially interested in the instruction for nursing and for exercises to use following childbirth.

POSTPARTUM EXERCISES

1. Practice the vaginal contractions learned during pregnancy. This restores the muscles of the birth canal to their former tightness and resiliency. If there have been stitches, they will heal more quickly, with less soreness.

2. Lie on your stomach from time to time with large pillows under the hips, and a small one under your ankles. The gravity of this position aids the uterus in returning to its normal place within the abdomen.

3. After returning home, once each day lie on your back, raise one leg ten inches off the ground without bending the knee, hold for a

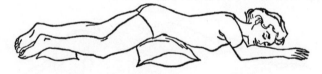

Fig. 13. Postpartum exercise two.

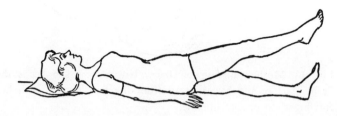

Fig. 14. Postpartum exercise three.

count of three, and lower slowly. Repeat with the other leg. Raise each leg two or three times each session, working up to ten times. This exercise will help restore the nice flat stomach of your high school days.

4. Practice good posture while sitting, standing, or walking, from the very first day.

BREAST-FEEDING INSTRUCTIONS

1. Breast-feed baby often during the first twenty-four hours. This will cause the uterus to contract firmly and help prevent hemorrhage. It will also loosen the colostrum (the creamy-looking secretion that appears before the milk comes in on about the third day), so that the milk will be "let down" more easily when it first appears. (Animals instinctively suckle their offspring shortly after birth.)

2. To breast-feed baby, place him on the bed beside you, lying on his side with his head tilted back ever so slightly. Lie on your side with the breast near his mouth. Compress his cheeks lightly between your thumb and middle finger so he will open his mouth, and insert all the brown part of the nipple into his mouth. (The nurses will be glad to help you at first.)

3. Let baby lie quietly beside you as he nurses. He should be handled as little as possible. With your index finger, keep the fleshy part of the breast pressed gently away from his nose, so he can breathe.

4. Breast-feed baby frequently the first day or two, a few minutes on each breast each time. This helps the milk come in more quickly and helps prevent engorgement and sore nipples.

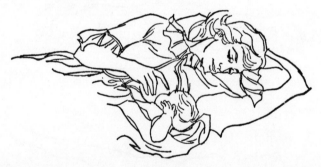

Fig. 15. Mother nursing her baby. Notice how she keeps the fleshy part of the breast away from the baby's nose with her forefinger, so he can breathe.

5. Baby may not get enough liquid to need burping the first few times, but after the milk comes in, this should be done after each feeding, and sometimes halfway through. Face him looking over your shoulder (be sure to support his head and neck) and pat his back gently. Or, sit him in your lap, leaning him forward slightly, cup his

chin in your hand to support his wobbly head, and pat his back until he "bubbles."

6. Baby will lose a few ounces of weight at first but will regain them rapidly when the milk begins to form (it looks thinner, more bluish than the colostrum, but don't worry—it's rich enough!). When the milk first appears, the breasts may become distended and overflow. Keep fresh, sterile pads (the hospital supplies them) over the nipples to absorb the excess milk. As the initial swelling of the breasts disappears, some mothers fear that they've "lost their milk," but the supply is only adjusting to the demand. As baby gets older, the amount of milk produced will increase to meet his demands.

7. Wash the nipples with water only, as soap is drying to the skin and may cause soreness and cracked nipples. If any soreness occurs, report it at once, and you will be given a bland ointment to help them heal quickly.

8. The breasts should always be well supported from beneath by a nursing brassiere, with no pressure across the breasts or nipples.

9. Whether breast-feeding baby in bed or sitting up in a chair, always lift him *to* the breast so there is no downward pull on it. If the breast is pulled down to the baby, it may lose its shape permanently.

10. Some doctors advise emptying the breast after each feeding. To do this, place the first joint of the forefinger just below, and the thumb just above, the outer edges of the brown area surrounding the nipple. Press these fingers gently in a scissors motion, at the same time pushing in toward the breast slightly. The milk will soon flow easily, and this is much more pleasant than the uncomfortable suction created by a breast pump, which is designed on the erroneous principle that a baby draws out the milk by suction. A baby doesn't actually "suck," but stimulates the "let-down" of the milk by the pressure of his gums, tongue, and palate around the nipple. This gentle squeezing action stimulates the milk flow, which is sometimes so rapid that the baby can hardly swallow fast enough at first!

11. If a premature baby is too weak to suckle, he still needs his mother's milk. The milk can be expressed manually directly into his mouth, or into a sterile container (after thoroughly scrubbing one's hands).

12. Relax and enjoy your baby.

Mary put down the folder, but before turning out her light, she gently pulled the baby's bed close to take a last peek at him, and to be sure—for the umpteenth time—that he was really breathing! He

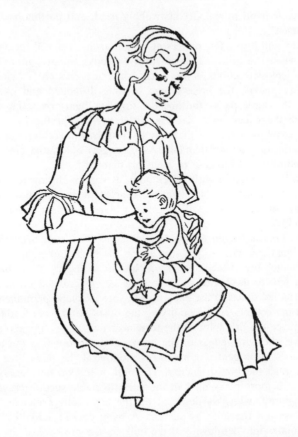

Fig. 16. Mother "burping" her baby. Notice how she cups his chin in her hand to support his wobbly head. This is a more effective way to bring up the "bubbles" than holding him against the shoulder, and it is less tiring to the mother.

was sleeping quietly, so she carefully pushed him back, turned over onto her stomach, relaxed as completely as she could, and had soon drifted into a peaceful, contented slumber. Her roommates were already asleep, and there were no sounds apart from the hushed rustling of normal night hospital activity.

Mary opened her eyes in the dark. Was that her baby? What

was that muffled sound? She lay very still, listening. Soon she realized that the sound she heard came from the bed next to hers. She sat up a moment, listening to the soft crying, and then slipped into her robe and slippers and tiptoed over to Janice's side.

"Janice?" she whispered anxiously. "Can I help? Please don't cry!"

Janice didn't answer, but turned her wet cheek toward Mary to indicate that she'd heard and appreciated Mary's concern. Mary took Janice's hand in her own and held it in the dark, tears of pity welling up in her own eyes, as Janice wept helplessly for several minutes.

"Please, Janice—don't cry any more," she pleaded.

"I can't—help it," Janice sobbed. "I'm a dope!" she berated herself, searching in her own mind for a reason for her unhappiness. "I've always wanted a little girl, and everyone's been so nice, but—" she burst into fresh sobs, "I can't help crying. I don't know what's the matter with me!"

Gradually Janice became quieter as Mary comforted her. There were deep, deep questions in Mary's heart as she stroked her companion's arm in the dark, wondering why Janice should be so unhappy.

"You have a beautiful baby, Janice," she suggested hopefully. "Nothing should take that happiness away from you."

Janice was quieter now. "I know," she said. Gradually she became aware of someone's else's need besides her own. "Mary, you're a gem!" she told her, "but you shouldn't be up and around in the middle of the night like this. You go on back to bed now. I'll be all right. And thank you so much." She pressed Mary's hand gratefully.

Mary took another peek at her baby. He was stirring, so she drew him close and laid him beside her. She needed the reassurance of his presence just now. As she helped his tiny rosebud mouth find satisfaction, Mary thought how grateful she was for her experience in giving him birth! That experience would be framed in her memory like a jewel, forever. She wouldn't have traded places with Janice for anything! As she caressed her baby's downy

head, she was so very happy that she'd had faith to believe that
God "giveth us richly all things to enjoy," not even excluding giving
birth to a baby.

Mary finished combing her hair, pinned a flower in place, and
returned to her bed, swinging her legs impatiently as she sat on the
edge of it waiting for her parents. "Mother! Dad!" she cried happily,
slipping down off the bed and hurrying forward to embrace them.

"Did you see Baby George before you came in?" she asked
breathlessly, not waiting for an answer as she perched back up on
the edge of the bed. "Isn't he a darling? Who does he look like?
Don't you think he looks like John? Of course, John doesn't have
such black hair."

"Just a minute, young lady," her father chided, holding up his
hand in mock dismay. He was pleased that she looked so well and
happy. "One question at a time please. So you think he looks like
John, eh? You're supposed to say he looks like *me*. Babies are supposed to resemble their grandparents more than their parents, you
know."

"I haven't decided who he looks like, but he's a darling!" her
mother smiled. "I can hardly wait till you bring him home, so I can
help spoil him!" Aside to Mary she whispered anxiously, "Doesn't
it make your stitches sore to sit on the edge of the bed like that?"

"But I don't have any stitches, Mother," Mary explained, "so I'm
not the least bit sore."

"You don't have any *stitches?*" Her mother sounded unbelieving.

Mary's dad realized that his womenfolk had momentarily forgotten him, so he wandered back out in the hall to take another
look at his new grandson. He read the small sign on the window
again:

Dr. Gordon, attending physician
Baby Thomas, boy
Seven pounds, nine ounces
Twenty-one inches
Born 10:58 P.M.   April 29

We men have to stick together, he said inwardly to his new grandson, as he studied the small face through the window, trying to find some resemblance in the tiny features—perhaps to himself!

"I didn't need any stitches," Mary was explaining to her mother. "And maybe you won't believe me, but it was the most *wonderful* experience! I can still feel how my baby's head slipped out and how his little body followed!" She sat transfixed in the happy memory for a moment. Her mother was silent, not understanding, but knowing from Mary's obvious happiness that her daughter was telling the truth.

"I'm truly glad for you, dear," she said earnestly, meaning every word.

Mary turned around and motioned to her friends. "Mother, I ought to introduce my roommates. This is Janice Wells—she has a little girl, the prettiest baby here."

"How do you do," Mary's mother said kindly, and Janice smiled acknowledgment.

"Down at the end is Elaine Dieple," Mary said, with a sweep of her arm. "She has five children now."

Mrs. Johnson and Elaine exchanged greetings. "This is a lovely room you have here, rocking chairs and all," Mary's mother told them. "Things have surely changed since I had my babies!"

"They've changed even since I started my family," Elaine agreed, "and for the better, I might add. It's so much nicer having our babies with us."

"Maybe this isn't such a new way after all," Mary's mother smiled. "I read in the paper last year that in maternity wards in the Congo, each mother's bed has a little basket at the foot of it. When reporters walked through one of the wards one day, not a single baby was in his basket! They were all in bed with their mothers!"

Mary's father walked into the room in time to hear her last comment. "So you're returning to the jungles to have your babies, are you?" he kidded them. He pulled up a chair and made himself comfortable.

"Not exactly, Dad," Mary laughed. "But we can learn a lot

from them." Then she asked him eagerly, "Did you decide who the baby looks like?"

"Yes, I did," he grinned mischievously.

"Who? Tell me!"

"Well, little mother," he teased her, "I think he favors the papa."

Chapter 16

For of Such Is the Kingdom of God

You must let little children come to me, and you must never stop them. The kingdom of heaven belongs to little children like these! Matt. 19:14 (Phillips translation).

"Aren't you about ready, Mary?" John called over his shoulder. "We're going to be late for church!"

"Just a minute! I'm changing the baby again." Mary was dressing the baby for the third time. "John," she reminded him, "you didn't take these blankets."

"More stuff!" he grumbled good-naturedly, coming back into the room to get them. "You'd think we were going to the North Pole!"

"A little baby *needs* a lot of things," Mary rationalized, deciding she'd better take an extra sweater for him, too. "Besides, Mom won't have anything at the house for him when we're there this afternoon."

John took the baby from Mary, and they hurried down the steps. A few moments later they reached the church.

"If it isn't the new baby!" Joanie greeted them, hurrying over to see him before they'd even entered. "Isn't he a darling," she cooed.

Every few steps someone else stopped the proud parents for a peek, until it seemed that they really would be late, even though they had arrived at the church on time.

157

Finally, they managed to slip away from the last eager admirer and seated themselves in the front pew with the other new mothers and fathers who were dedicating their babies on this Mother's Day Sunday. The thoughts of all the parents were hushed, after the bustling of preparation, by the familiar tones of the hymn, "Praise God from Whom All Blessings Flow." As the majestic voice of the organ crescendoed the familiar melody into the sanctuary, it hung vibrating in radiant eloquence in the reverent air.

All blessings! John thought, looking at the tiny bundle he was holding in his arms. Glancing at Mary out of the corner of his eye, he thought she had never looked more beautiful. God had surely been good to him! Gradually he became aware of the preacher saying something and that the other parents were rising to their feet. He stood up, too. Each father held his baby, and each mother held a red rose that had been placed in her hands.

The dedication ceremony was short and simple. To everyone's surprise (and to the disappointment of a few people in the audience), not a baby cried. Afterward, some of the parents took their babies to the nursery, but since George was sleeping soundly, John and Mary simply moved a few pews farther back with him. The new grandmother hovered near, more than anxious to have the opportunity to take him out and rock him if he cried.

"With every great blessing," Pastor Dirkson told his congregation earnestly, "comes great responsibility. This is especially true of the blessing of a new baby brought into a home. For, as parents have, in renunciation of themselves, carefully prepared for the physical arrival of their child, so they must, in renunciation of all selfish desires, continue to give of themselves in the years to come, for his spiritual, as well as his physical, welfare.

"For a child is much more than a physical being. He is also an immortal soul! And as it is the Creator's plan to make possible, through a father and a mother, the physical life of a child, so it is His plan to make possible, through their dedicated lives, the child's awareness of and obedience to Himself.

"For you see, the Bible teaches that God is like the first persons that a little child knows—his father and his mother! In the gentleness of his father's strength the child is to learn of the pity of a mighty God for the weakness of man, as the Psalmist describes it:

> Like as a father pitieth his children, so the Lord pitieth them that fear him.

"From the loving providence of his father in meeting all his material needs, the child is to learn to trust also in the providence of his heavenly Father, to whom Jesus said:

> What man is there of you, whom if his son ask bread, will he give him a stone? . . .
>
> How much more shall your Father which is in heaven give good things to them that ask him?

"From the constancy of his mother's steadfast love, which is never forgetful of his needs, the child is to learn of the greater constancy of the love of God:

> Can a woman forget her sucking child, that she should not have compassion on the son of her womb? yea, they may forget, yet will I not forget thee!

"And from his mother's tender comforting, as she soothes away his tears in his times of unhappiness, he is to learn of the loving God who bears all our sorrows, and who can restore to us joy for any trouble, for the Bible says: 'As one whom his mother comforteth, so will I comfort you.'

"As the child grows older, both parents share in training him in a growing awareness of his responsibility to God:

> The fear of the Lord is the beginning of knowledge: . . .
>
> My son, hear the instruction of thy father,
> And forsake not the law of thy mother.

"And both parents share in the daily teaching of the words of God found in Scripture to the child:

Thou shalt teach them diligently unto thy children, and shalt talk of them when thou sittest in thine house, and when thou walkest by the way, and when thou liest down, and when thou risest up.

"Thus we realize that it was God's plan, when He ordained that new human beings should not come into the world as solitary creatures, but should be set 'in families,' that through this means they are to be brought into fellowship with the Creator. What a grave responsibility parents receive, with the gift from God of a tiny baby!

"But in the harmony and self-giving love of a godly home, in which a child is brought up by his father and his mother to know and trust the Creator who made him, we see the perfect wisdom of the unfolding pattern of God's design: father, mother, child!"

Part II

Chapter 17

Evidences From Anthropology

PRIMITIVE LABORS

There are two common misconceptions concerning childbirth among primitive peoples. The first is that "all primitive labors are painless"; the second is that "all womankind suffers agony in childbirth." Neither assumption is correct.

In every culture there are instances of difficulty such as abnormal presentation, disproportion, or uterine inertia. Attempts to relieve these conditions in primitive societies have frequently led to unbelievably cruel treatment of the suffering woman in order to force the child from her body. These attempts usually resulted in her death and in the death of her child. Furthermore, primitive women are ignorant of the physiology of conception, pregnancy, and birth. They are also ignorant of the basic rules of good nutrition and personal hygiene, nor have they been taught how to relax during labor.

Obviously, "natural" childbirth is not "primitive" childbirth, as some have contended. The woman interested in a natural birth has the advantage of adequate prenatal training, and she has access to all present-day scientific aids if she has an abnormal condition that presents a problem. Analgesia, anesthesia, incision of the perineum, extraction of the baby by forceps, Cesarean delivery, blood transfusions, and antibiotics are all available in the event that she needs them.

The astonishing fact remains, however, that despite all the disadvantages and the ignorant superstitions which surround it, normal childbirth for women in most of the primitive societies was shorter, easier and accepted more matter-of-factly, whether or not a certain amount of discomfort accompanied it. On this point, most anthropologists agree:

> It is a strange thing that most of the anxiety over the crises of childbirth comes before the event, not at it. Magic, ritual, and tabu dominate the prenatal period, yet when the moment of birth is reached, the obstetrical problems are in normal cases handled with matter-of-fact effectiveness free of mumbo jumbo.[1]

Obviously, a careful study of the environmental and cultural factors that have contributed to easier childbirth among other peoples is useful. It is helpful to realize, for example, that the primitive woman developed flexibility in her pelvic and hip joints by crouching by her little fire to prepare the evening meal, and that she increased muscle tone and breath control in her long walk to the village well. These things made a tremendous difference to the facility and comfort with which she delivered her child, and her instinctive suckling of her newborn soon after the birth helped protect her from hemorrhaging.

Examples of easy deliveries in the more primitive cultures are numerous. Margaret Mead relates the following personal experience:

> . . . One consideration in choosing that particular site was that Bangwin, our next-door neighbor, had a pregnant wife, and births are very hard to see in primitive society, where babies are likely to be born at 2 A.M. or when the mother is out fishing. True, in the end Bangwin's baby too was born when Tshamwole was out fishing.[2]

In a very different part of the world from Polynesia, Eskimo women often gave birth while migrating across the ice and snow. After the birth, the mother slipped the baby beneath her clothing at her bosom to keep it warm and resumed her journey. A very recent example of this was a fifteen-year-old Laplander who delivered her own twins one bitterly cold day while she was alone in the woods. She then walked *fifteen miles* to the nearest community, carrying her babies wrapped in fur bags. A doctor who examined them said that mother and babies were in excellent condition.

Thousands of additional examples could be given to demonstrate that *there is no anthropological evidence to support the theological dogma that women of all cultures have universally regarded childbirth as an "illness" or a "curse."*

On the contrary, it is probable that the joy of motherhood, which follows the satisfying orgasm of the birth experience, has enabled women in many cultures to adapt themselves successfully to unfortunate social conditions. A non-Christian woman from India expressed this philosophy by saying that bearing children had satisfied a deep personal need in her life, and that she believed that nature had been kinder to women than to men!

CULTURAL DIFFERENCES

While it is true that women in most cultures have accepted the birth process matter-of-factly, Western culture is not the only one which deviates from this attitude. In societies where women attempt to identify themselves with the men, childbirth and motherhood are not well regarded. Among the warlike Aztecs with their highly developed culture, for example, there is evidence that the women disliked their role intensely. Among the Manus of New Guinea this was also true: the sex act was conducted prudishly, with a sense of shame, and all a woman's distinctive creative functions were undervalued.

In still other cultures quite the opposite is seen, and men have sought to identify themselves in some way with the birth process. Among the Basques in Spain the women would get up and go back to work after the birth of a child, while their husbands went to bed for a period of time. This quaint custom is called the couvade, and it is found in many parts of the world. The practice of couvade has been found in South American cultures, in African tribes, in south India, in China, and among the Ainus of Japan.

In some cultures the mother remained separated for a period of

time after childbirth, whether or not the father is also "lying-in."
Her separation was usually akin to that required because of menstrual taboos which existed in that particular society rather than to
any physiological inability to go back to her normal tasks as other
primitive women do. Many cultures have regarded menstruation
superstitiously and treated it with religious restrictions. In these
societies, the normal lochial discharge following childbirth has been
equated with menstruation and the woman is subjected to the same
restrictions.

The Mountain Arapesh tribe of New Guinea provides good examples of menstrual taboos and a type of couvade:

> Men have to stay away from the edge of the village where
> women bear their children, and wonder, with anguished curiosity
> that will never be satisfied, what it is like to bear children. Both
> boys and girls have to guard their growth so that they will be
> good parents. They will both be depleted by parenthood, a man
> no less than a woman. "You should have seen what a fine-
> looking man he was before he had all those children!" . . . To
> the female periodicities, both men and women adjust. During
> menstruation the woman rests in a small, badly built shelter over
> the edge of the hillside, and the man must fend for himself,
> care for the children, and abstain from entering his yam-garden,
> from which she is debarred. So during pregnancy he shares her
> taboos, and after child-birth he lies beside his newly-delivered
> wife, resting from the labour, from the hard work of child-
> bearing, which ages a man as much as it does a woman![3]

ANCIENT HEBREW CULTURE

The first chapter of Exodus reveals that the women in Moses'
day gave birth easily and often without assistance. Moses himself
was born to his mother without her receiving assistance, or his
presence would have been known (Exodus 2:2). The Hebrew midwives explained to Pharaoh that the Hebrew women were not like
the indolent women of the Egyptian court and were often delivered
of the children before the midwife could get to them.

The harder Pharaoh made the Hebrews work, the stronger they
became, and the more easily did the women give birth to their

babies. Although the statement of the midwives was made to explain to Pharaoh why they had not destroyed the male infants of
the Hebrews, it must have been credible or it would not have been
accepted.

Because the midwives feared God, "he gave them families"
(Exodus 1:21, RSV). In other words, God *blessed* these women
whose lives were committed to helping other women in childbirth
by giving them the privilege of giving birth to many children themselves!

In Exodus 1:16 mention is made of a "stool" or "birthstool"
(RSV) which the Hebrew women supposedly used when giving
birth. But the Hebrews did not ordinarily use "stools" or "chairs"
unless they were wealthy or persons of importance. Even in Christ's
day people ordinarily reclined even at meals.

The Hebrew word translated "birthstool" is *ovnayim,* which
means literally "two stones." The manner in which these stones were
used is not certain, but mention of them indicates that the Hebrew
births frequently took place as the women were working in the
fields, as is common in other primitive cultures. The Levitical law
requiring women to be "separated" for "purification" following
childbirth had not yet been made, and the women probably resumed
their tasks after the birth of the child.

A woman might have used these stones to lean against for support as she crouched, or knelt, to bear her child. Or, if someone
was supporting her, she might have pushed against them with her
feet to aid her expulsive efforts. But however she used them, it is
highly unlikely that she sat on them, as the translation "stool" implies. The Hebrew woman usually crouched on her heels to give
birth (as in I Samuel 4:19), while another woman knelt between
her legs to receive the child onto her waiting lap (as in Genesis
30:3).

THE EARLY CHRISTIAN ERA

There were two basic influences on the cultural attitude of the
first-century Christians toward childbirth: the influences of the
Hebrew and of the Greek cultures.

The Jews had a high regard for motherhood. Multiple births were considered an event of special honor to a woman, rather than being regarded with superstition as in many primitive cultures. As has been noted, in the Pentateuch childbirth is described as a simple process. In Isaiah and Jeremiah, prophets of a leisure-class court society, some illustrations are given that refer to exhausting labors. However, there is no indication that this was the case among the peasants of Palestine in Christ's day. Our Lord Himself was born with no mention made of anyone assisting His mother. Indeed, Mary had undertaken a lengthy journey on the eve of her pregnancy, as is commonly done among primitives and peasants, who think nothing of giving birth to their babies en route.

Jewish mothers loved their children dearly, and always breast-fed their own babies, a precious function to them. Moses' mother was reluctant to let an Egyptian woman wet-nurse her son, and even prostitutes breast-fed their own children. Most babies were fed at the breast for two years or more, and later Talmudic regulation forbade a woman to remarry until two years after the birth of her last child, lest the orphan be deprived of her full attention.

Among the Greeks of the pre-Christian era, medicine had reached a high state, which was maintained from the time of Hippocrates until the Roman conquest, when the more barbaric Romans then copied much of the Greek culture. Although the Greeks had no scruples about men attending women in labor (nor did the Jews), most deliveries were conducted by midwives. Physicians were called only in difficult cases. Births must have been relatively simple, since so little mention is made of obstetrics in the medical literature. The Greek woman lived an active, outdoor life and wore loose and free-flowing clothes, especially in pregnancy. The importance of physical preparation for childbirth was recognized, and Lycurgus, the ancient lawgiver, instituted exercises for growing girls so that they would have easy labors and produce healthier offspring.

The midwives had high standards of practice and were required to be scrupulously clean, honest, and industrious. As with the

Jews, cleanliness was important, and the story of Achilles, who was plunged into the river Styx after his birth by his mother, is well known. He was completely washed except for his heel, where his mother was holding him!

But in contrast to the Jews, the Greeks practiced abortion and infanticide freely, and weak-looking newborn babies were destroyed without compunction. The Jews used abortion for therapeutic reasons, such as to protect a mother who had suffered in childbirth from having a similar experience, but they looked aghast at any form of infanticide.

The early Church retained the Jewish regard for motherhood and was familiar as well with the Greek teachings of good midwifery. The writings of the earliest Church fathers demonstrates their great respect for a woman's creative functions of pregnancy, childbirth, nursing, and motherhood, as the following examples illustrate:

Ignatius (A.D. 30–107) writes:

> Children, obey your parents, and have an effection for them, as workers together with God for your birth into the world. . . . Husbands, love your wives, as fellow-servants of God, as your own body, as the partners of your life, and your co-adjutors in the procreation of children.[4]

Clement of Rome (A.D. 30–100) demonstrates the wisdom of God, the great "Creator" and "Designer of the universe," by illustrating His providence in making mankind male and female:

> Moreover, the female form, and the cavity of the womb, most suitable for receiving and cherishing and vivifying the germ . . . in which the foetus being placed, is kept and cherished. . . . Who will not, from all these things, acknowledge the operation of reason, and the wisdom of the Creator?[5]

Clement of Alexandria (A.D. 153–217):

> Let us . . . understand that the virtue of man and woman is the same. . . . one church, one temperance, one modesty; their food is common, marriage an equal yoke. . . .[6]

As far as respects human nature, the woman does not possess one nature, and the man exhibit another, but the same: so also with righteousness, and every other virtue. . . . Undoubtedly it stands to reason that some difference should exist between each of them, in virtue of which one is male and the other female. Pregnancy, and parturition, accordingly, belong to woman. . . . As then there is sameness, as far as respects the soul, she will attain to the same virtue; but as there is difference as respects the peculiar construction of the body, she is destined for childbearing.[7]

DARK CLOUDS ON THE HORIZON

Midwifery customs of Roman civilization during the early Christian era were almost identical with those of the earlier Greeks. But Roman civilization became far more dissolute. By the time the early Church had come into existence Roman morals were already in a rapid state of decline. Roman rulers set the example, and the masses soon followed suit:

Both Julius Caesar and Augustus led dissolute lives. Caligula kept a brothel in his palace and by taxing the keepers of the *lupanaria* he was able to derive a substantial income from their infamous calling. Nero not only visited the houses of the prostitutes and dined in public with a crowd of these creatures, but he also founded on the shores of the Gulf of Naples, houses of ill-fame, which he filled with the most abandoned women. Commodus was surrounded by no less than three hundred maidens. But perhaps none reached the depths of depravity sounded by the Emperor Claudius Tiberius, whose amours at Capreae cannot be described.

Morally the wives of these Emperors were often little better than their husbands. Agrippina used to leave the palace of the Caesars and go to the brothels of Rome where she would spend the night in debauchery. . . .[8]

The influx of Greek slaves into Rome freed women in the leisure classes from their normal responsibilities, so that they could spend their time in sex indulgence. There were many more men than women, which increased the temptations to debauchery. But to offset this abnormal sexual activity, induced abortions became so common that some Roman leaders feared the race would die out. There was one full year in a city along the Tiber when not a single birth took place!

> Plautus, the Latin playwright, described it [abortion] as a natural step in the life of the Roman woman. Terence, foreseeing the consequence of excess, moaned over its frequency, Juvenal grimly remarked that the Roman wives no longer had any lying-in; Ovid, perhaps facetiously, referred to a league for abortion that was organized by the Roman women.[9]

Rome had become one of those societies in which women consider pregnancy and childbirth a nuisance and an ordeal: Furthermore, the Roman mother refused to breast-feed her own child, turning it over to wet nurses after the birth. Following his weaning, he was reared by Greek slaves rather than by his mother.

What was the reaction of the infant Church to all this? As might be expected, many Christians overreacted—to the extent that they regarded *all* sexual intercourse as sinful, and the "ordeal" of childbirth was considered the inevitable judgment of God upon the woman who had indulged herself. Evidence of this morbid attitude appears by the second century A.D., and continues to develop:

Tertullian (A.D. 145–220 or 240):

> Therefore when, through the will of God, the husband is deceased, the marriage likewise, by the will of God, deceases. Why should *you* restore what God has put an end to? Why do you, by repeating the servitude of maternity, spurn the liberty which is offered you? . . .[10]

> Marrying, let us be overtaken by the last day, like Sodom and Gomorrah; that day when "woe" pronounced over "such as are with child and giving suck" shall be fulfilled, that is, over the married and the incontinent: for from marriage result wombs, and breasts, and infants![11]

Cyprian (A.D. 200–258):

> Do you wish to know what ill the virtue of continence avoids, what good it possesses? "I will multiply," says God to the

woman, "thy sorrows and thy groanings; and in sorrow shalt thou bring forth children and thy desire shall be to thy husband, and he shall rule over thee." You are free from this sentence. You do not fear the sorrows and the groans of women. You have no fear of child-bearing; nor is your husband lord over you. . . .[12]

Jerome (A.D. 346–420), on a pilgrimage to the Holy Land, was accompanied by a woman named Paula, and one can see the contempt in which motherhood was held by the Church in her example:

> She resisted the entreaties of all her relatives. In vain her youngest daughter, Rufina, who had recently been affianced, implored her with tears to await her approaching marriage; in vain her little son Toxotius uplifted from the shore his suppliant hands. Paula raised heavenwards her tearless eyes, and, turning her back to the shore, *ignored her motherhood to prove her saintlessness.* (Italics added.)[13]

What the young Church did not realize was that in its reaction to Roman licentiousness and abortions, it was unconsciously absorbing the Roman contempt for marriage, childbearing, and motherhood. *Thus the Church became infiltrated with the Roman attitude toward the nuisance of childbearing and motherhood which was in direct contrast to the continuing Jewish concept of the blessedness of marriage and maternity.*

In addition, the Gnostic belief that the physical body was evil was accepted by some early Christian writers. Because of this erroneous belief in the sinful nature of the physical body, women, because their very bodies excited the physical desires of men, were thought to be deserving of God's special judgment.

This morbid attitude continued through medieval times. Knowledge of good midwifery almost vanished, and deliveries were frequently attended by untrained, superstitious old women. Physicians were forbidden by the Church to be present at the scene of birth, and the midwife had nothing to rely upon except her own "magic." For fifteen hundred years the advances in obstetric knowledge that had been made by the Greeks and Romans were lost to the world.

Because the midwives frequently used ritualistic chants and oblations in aiding a birth, they were often accused of witchcraft. This occasioned such inquiries as:

> . . . whether you know anye that doe use charmes, sorcery, enchantments, invocations, circles, witchcrafts, soothsayings or any like crafts or imaginations invented by the Devyle and especially in the tyme of women's travyle.[14]

Of course, from time to time there were women whose midwifery ability was excellent, but they appear briefly in medieval history, and their warnings against abuses were unheeded. The only medical advances of any consequence during this time were among the Arabs and the Jews. The Jewish doctor was never restricted from attending women in labor, nor was he forbidden to destroy the unborn child if the life of the mother was at stake, because the Jews believed that the infant did not become a "soul" until he had drawn his first breath. Evidence for this was taken from the account of Adam's creation in Genesis 2:7:

> And the Lord God . . . breathed into his nostrils the breath of life; and man became a living soul.

The Church forbade any form of abortion under any circumstances, allowing the mother to die as well as the child. The agony of the dying woman, unable to deliver her infant, was considered to be God's judgment upon her for the sin of Eve.

THE RENAISSANCE—AND CATASTROPHE!

With the revival of learning the outlook for the woman in labor seemed optimistic. Discoveries were being made in human anatomy and physiology, a greater number of hospitals were being provided, and male physicians were once again reluctantly permitted to attend births.

But it soon became apparent that the parturient woman was in a far more serious plight than in medieval times, for a strange and terrible malady appeared more and more frequently. Puerperal fever (a septic poisoning) attacked women after childbirth, taking them through feverish, racking agony to almost certain death. By 1652 the disease had assumed epidemic proportions, and it raged across Europe unabated for the next two hundred years.

In 1795 Dr. Gordon of Aberdeen, Scotland, announced that he felt certain the disease was of infectious origin, but other doctors ignored him. Oliver Wendell Holmes, the American physician, wrote a treatise in 1843 called "Puerperal Fever as a Private Pestilence," in which he claimed that the disease was contagious and that the doctors themselves were transmitting it. His warning was likewise ignored. It remained for Dr. Philipp Semmelweiss, an Austrian physician, to prove conclusively the direct relationship between the attending physician's lack of personal cleanliness and the resulting puerperal infection of the mother. He was mocked by the medical profession, and died before his discovery was really accepted.

Only a hundred years ago a physician would frequently go directly from dissecting a corpse to assist a woman in labor, *without even washing his hands in water!* The doctors themselves were infecting the mothers and causing their deaths.

Contrast this practice with the Jewish regard for cleanliness taught by Moses and enforced by Jewish law. This was especially true in regard to disposal of the dead, after which one was required to bathe, wash his clothes, and remain "unclean" the rest of the day. Without knowing the principles of sanitation, such observances nevertheless protected the Hebrew mother, and the nation as well, from infections of this origin.

The mortality rate at the lying-in division of the Vienna General Hospital where Dr. Semmelweiss worked was staggering. But in 1847 he tried an experiment: all physicians under his authority were required to wash their hands in a chloride of lime solution before entering the labor rooms, and the incidence of the fever dropped sharply. Even so, he was labeled the "Pesth fool" (Pesth was his birthplace) by other physicians, and eventually he was forced to leave Vienna. He continued his work at the Pesth hospital, where he could get more co-operation.

In the cities of Norway, in Vienna, in Paris, Kiev, and Berlin, physicians practiced midwifery on cadavers, left the corpses when called to a woman in labor, and transmitted cadaveric poisoning to her because they had not even washed. In the crowded labor wards, after examining one woman internally, they simply wiped the blood and pus from their hands onto their waistcoats, and proceeded to the next patient, thrusting their filthy hands into her birth canal to see how the labor was progressing.

> There was always a surplus of motherless children. Vienna's mother and child mortality was enormous. But the world was used to such deaths. There were years when in Paris the Hôtel Dieu lost more than half the women who gave birth there. There were *four years when at the University of Jena not a mother left the hospital alive.* (Italics added.)[15]

In 1847 there were so many maternal deaths at the Kiev hospital that the hospital was closed. The director, "heavy with a sense of personal guilt," committed suicide. In 1854, however, Semmelweiss's theory was well proven in the hospital in Pesth where he delivered the mothers, but it was rejected throughout Europe.

> In the seven years since the discovery of the cause and the simple prevention of childbed fever had been clearly announced, at least seventy thousand and perhaps a third of a million women had died of childbed fever. As to the babies, there was no counting![16]

With such terrible suffering connected with childbirth for over two hundred years, is it any wonder that Bible translators and scholars began interpreting Genesis 3:16 as meaning *"suffering* in childbirth"? This pain and death, which women feared and men could not understand, was said to be due to the "hand of God" punishing womankind—the curse of "pain" on Eve!

Yet men could not escape their own sense of guilt over the staggering number of childbirth deaths, and the Puritan concept of the shamefulness of intercourse pervaded Europe. We are not entirely free of this sense of wrong even today. Less than twenty years ago the eminent Bible scholar, the Reverend J. B. Phillips, showed the inconsistency of some Christians' thinking about God in relation to sex and other physical matters:

> We may, for instance, admire the ascetic ultra-spiritual type which appears to have "a mind above" food, sexual attraction, and material comfort, for example. But if in forming a picture of the Holiness of God we are simply enlarging this spirituality and asceticism to the "nth" degree we are forced to some peculiar conclusions. Thus we may find ourselves readily able to imagine God's interest in babies (for are they not "little bits of Heaven"?) yet unable to imagine His approval, let alone design, of the acts which led to their conception![17]

The common mistaken belief in Western cultures that a woman must be punished for giving a man pleasure in intercourse and that God's whole plan for the reproduction of the human race is a morbid one, was strikingly illustrated in Leo Tolstoy's writings. Notice, for example, Prince Andrew's feelings of guilt after his wife Lise dies in childbirth:

> Prince Andrew ran to the door; the scream ceased and he heard the wail of an infant. . . . Suddenly he realized the joyful significance of that wail; tears choked him, and leaning his elbows on the window sill he began to cry, sobbing like a child. . . . He went into his wife's room. She was lying dead, in the same position he had seen her in five minutes before. . . . "I love you all, and have done no harm to anyone; and *what have you done to me?"* said her charming, pathetic, dead face. . . . Prince Andrew felt that something gave way in his soul and that he *was guilty of a sin that he could neither remedy nor forget.* (Italics added.)[18]

Notes

1. E. A. Hoebel, *Man in the Primitive World* (New York: McGraw-Hill, 1958), p. 372. See also Palmer Findley, M.D., *Priests of Lucina, The Story of Obstetrics* (Boston: Little, Brown, 1939).

2. Margaret Mead, *Male and Female* (New York: Morrow, 1949), p. 42. Reprinted by permission.
3. Mead, *Male and Female*, pp. 101, 102, 1069. Reprinted by permission.
4. "Epistle of Ignatius to the Philadelphians," Chap. IV, in *The Ante-Nicene Fathers* (Grand Rapids: Eerdmans, 1951), Vol. 1, p. 81.
5. "Recognitions of Clement," Book VIII, Chap. XXXII, in *The Ante-Nicene Fathers,* Vol. VIII, p. 173, 174.
6. "The Instructor," Book I, Chap. IV, in *The Ante-Nicene Fathers,* Vol. II, p. 211.
7. "The Stromata, or Miscellanies," Book IV, Chap. VIII, in *The Ante-Nicene Fathers,* Vol. II, pp. 419 ff.
8. Roy P. Finney, M.D., *The Story of Motherhood* (New York: Liveright, 1937), pp. 42, 43.
9. A. J. Rongy, M.D., *Childbirth: Yesterday and Today* (New York: Emerson, 1937), pp. 162, 163.
10. "To His Wife," Book I, Chap. VII, in *The Ante-Nicene Fathers,* Vol. IV, p. 43.
11. "Exhortations to Chastity," Chap. IX, in *The Ante-Nicene Fathers,* Vol. IV, p. 55.
12. "The Treatises of Cyprian," Treatise II, in *The Ante-Nicene Fathers,* Vol. V, p. 436.
13. F. W. Farrar, *Lives of the Fathers* (Edinburgh: Black, 1889), Vol. II, pp. 302, 303.
14. Quoted by Rongy in *Childbirth: Yesterday and Today,* p. 86.
15. Morton Thompson, *The Cry and the Covenant* (Garden City, N.Y.: Doubleday, 1949), p. 107.
16. *Ibid.,* p. 108.
17. J. B. Phillips, *Your God Is Too Small* (New York: Macmillan, 1954), p. 38.
18. Leo Tolstoy, *War and Peace* (New York: Simon and Schuster, 1942), pp. 347–54.

Chapter 18

Theological Considerations

INTRODUCTION

That it is possible to give birth without pain has now been demonstrated for over fifty years. This has given occasion for materialistic Russia (which now uses the natural childbirth method almost exclusively) to call the Bible false and to scoff at Christians for believing childbirth pain is inevitable due to the "curse of Eve."

It is not the Bible that degrades womanhood in this manner and labels childbearing a curse. Rather, it is this *interpretation* of the Bible which is at fault, just as the interpretation of our forefathers was faulty when they used the Bible to "prove" that the earth was flat. The Bible is not a scientific text, to be abused in this manner, and one does not either "prove" or "disprove" natural childbirth by "using" the Bible.

But if Christianity is relevant to every experience of life, then it is relevant to childbirth. And if the Bible provides broad, underlying principles by which we may examine any philosophy concerning life, then it is imperative for us to examine the philosophy of natural childbirth in the light of these principles. And to do this, we must first discover exactly what the Bible does say about childbirth.

It must be realized at the outset of this survey that it is beyond the purpose of this book to suggest the sources of any text, such as the Genesis account of the Creation and Fall, or to suggest

178

whether the record is to be taken as literal, allegorical, or mythological. The purposes here are three:

1. To determine as closely as possible the accurate meaning of the original Hebrew words.

2. To determine whether or not the English translators have consistently translated these words accurately (the inspiration of the Bible surely cannot be defined as meaning that every *translation* of it, into any language, is without error).

3. To suggest how inconsistent renderings of certain words have helped to create and maintain the negative philosophy toward the birth process that is so embedded in our culture.

Since this book is primarily for the lay reader, the word *etsev* is used for either *etsev* or its cognates. This same principle applies as well to all other Hebrew, Greek, or Latin words used.

Also, since frequent mention is made of the Jewish Septuagint, Mishnah, and Talmud, the following brief definitions are given as an aid to lay readers:

1. The Septuagint is a translation of the Hebrew Old Testament into Greek by Hebrew scholars, during the third and second centuries B.C.

2. The Mishnah was the name given to the Jewish Oral Law, the "tradition of the elders," which was at first passed down from generation to generation by word of mouth. After this Oral Law was written down in the third century A.D. it was called the Mishnah, and it consists of detailed instructions developed by the rabbis on how to observe the Law of Moses.

3. The Talmud is composed of the Mishnah and an interpretation of each of its passages by rabbis. It was written down during the fourth to sixth centuries A.D. Its interpretive approaches are both allegorical and literal.

ETSEV AND THE "CURSE OF EVE"

It has already been noted in Chapter 7 that *etsev* refers primarily to the emotions. Rabbi Hirsch explains this aspect of the word as follows:

> 1. *Etsev:* only a *mental* pain and hurt feelings or worry. . . .
> The root is . . . a modification of . . . "forsaken," . . . leaving
> something against one's will . . . so that *etsev* is the feeling that
> we have to give something up that we would have liked to keep,
> or to have attained: renouncing, forgoing (I Kings 1:6—"David
> had never asked his son to give anything up.") . . . Until then
> Man knew no wrong, and no renunciation. But now for Man
> nature is no longer at one with his wishes as it was previ-
> ously, he must wrest everything from her, and only by re-
> nunciation, by giving up one thing, one enjoyment, can he attain
> another.[1]

In our English translations of the Bible *etsev* is frequently given as
"labor," or "toil." Although this might not be accurate in the strict-
est sense, it is so closely related to the concept of "giving of oneself" that it seems to be a legitimate translation. It appears this way
in Genesis 5:29, where Lamech says of his son Noah:

> This same shall comfort us concerning our work and *toil* (**etsev**)
> of our hands, because of the ground which the Lord hath cursed.

Etsev is also translated as "toil" in Proverbs 5:10; Proverbs
10:22 (marginal reading); Isaiah 58:3, etc. Notice how it is used
in the RSV in Proverbs 14:23 and Psalm 127:2. To be consistent,
it should also be translated as "toil" in I Chronicles 4:9. Interest-
ingly enough, this verse is the *only* one in the entire Bible which
uses *etsev* in connection with the birth of a child. Furthermore, the
mother says that this was her favorite child, because she gave birth
to him with *toil* (**etsev**):

> And Jabez was more honourable than his brethren: and his
> mother called his name Jabez [meaning "height"], saying, Be-
> cause I bare him with *etsev*.

After discussing *etsev*, Rabbi Hirsch makes it very plain that in
the interpretation of the third chapter of Genesis, Judaism and
Christianity part company, for it is here that the Christian doctrine
of original sin and the consequent need for a Saviour, begin. He
says:

Mankind is in no manner whatsoever placed under a ban for his first disobedience. . . . Still today, every human child comes from the hand of God as pure as Adam did, still today every child is born to mankind as pure as an angel. This is one of the cardinal points of Jewish life and of the essential Jewish nature. . . . Certainly, through this sin, all the descendants of Adam have inherited the task of having to live in a world which no longer smiles benevolently in harmony with them, but that is just because the same sin is constantly being repeated. . . . But that . . . *something else* is required other than the possibility which everyone possesses to *elevate himself* up to faithful fulfillment of duty, against that belief Judaism raises the most vehement protest. For that, no dead, and no resurrected intermediary is necessary. This is taught by the whole of Jewish history.

Adam could well have railed at his wife for the loss of Paradise and he calls her by the loveliest calling of Woman! Man had been allotted renunciation, Woman had been allotted renunciation, but the purpose for which Woman had been given renunciation was the higher; *she had become the savior from death, the dispenser of life, in her the immortality of mankind took refuge.*[2] (Italics added.)

Clearly, then, the origins of the belief that all womankind is under a curse in childbirth could not have existed in Judaism, as some have claimed. The Jews, in placing woman in the position of "savior from death, the dispenser of life," put her in the place of our Lord Jesus Christ. The origins of the "curse" obviously come later, in the third and fourth centuries, as has already been outlined in the previous chapter.

Rabbi Hirsch's interpretation of the Genesis passage is not new among the Jews, for Josephus, the Jewish historian who lived and wrote in the first century A.D., also points out that since Adam's time, mankind no longer lives in a world which "smiles benevolently in harmony with them":

God said, "Nay, I had decreed for you to live a life of bliss, unmolested by all ill, with no care to fret your souls; all things that contribute to enjoyment and pleasure were, through my providence, to spring up for you spontaneously, without toil or distress of yours. Blessed with these gifts, old age would not soon have overtaken you and your life would have been long. But now thou hast flouted this my purpose by disobeying my commands.[3]

A second-century Christian, Irenaeus, writes prior to the time when the teaching developed that the physical body was evil, that the actual "curse" of Genesis 3 was only upon the ground and the serpent, and that God showed compassion toward the sinners:

> For God is neither devoid of power nor of justice, who has afforded help to Man, and restored him to His own liberty. It was for this reason, too, that immediately after Adam had transgressed, as the Scripture relates, He pronounced no curse against Adam personally, but against the ground . . . But the curse in all its fulness fell upon the serpent, which had beguiled them. . . . For God detested him who had led Man astray, but by degrees and little by little, He showed compassion to him who had been beguiled.[4]

The word *adam* that Irenaeus uses here, is the generic name meaning "Adam and Eve," and was so used by the Jews as well as the Christians:

> All the races of men are descended from a single pair, to whom with their posterity God gave the generic name Man (Hebrew *adam*). That God made from one (ancestor) every race of men to settle all over the face of the earth in times and bounds of His appointment, was universal Jewish doctrine.[5]

THE BLESSING OF CHILDBIRTH IN THE OLD AND NEW TESTAMENTS

That bearing children was considered a blessing from God in Bible times is abundantly evident. Take the story of Leah, for example, which tells how God blessed her with many children in order to compensate for Rachel's being the favored wife:

> And when the Lord saw that Leah was hated, he opened her womb: but Rachel was barren. And Leah conceived, and bare

a son, and she called his name Reuben: for she said, Surely
the Lord hath looked upon my affliction. . . . (Gen. 29:31 ff.).

Godly Hannah was also blessed for her faith, not only by the
birth of Samuel but with five other sons and daughters as well:

> And the Lord visited Hannah, so that she conceived, and bare
> three sons and two daughters. (I Sam. 2:21.)

Other passages confirm that childbirth was a blessing, as in
Genesis 29:25; Deuteronomy 7:13; 28:11, 12; Ruth 4:13; Psalm
127:3, and many others. That it was considered a judgment of God
not to bear children can be demonstrated from verses like:

> Give them, O Lord: what wilt thou give? give them a miscarry-
> ing womb and dry breasts . . . [for] all their wickedness. . . . (Hos.
> 9:14.)

The happy comments of Bible mothers is further evidence of the
blessedness that they considered motherhood to be. Read the comments of Sarah, Genesis 21:6, 7; Rebecca, Genesis 25:21, 22, who
took her worries about her pregnancy to God in prayer; Leah,
Genesis 29:31–35 and 30:17–21; Manoah's wife, Judges 13:2, 3,
whose spiritual perception was keener than her husband's at this
time; Hannah, I Samuel 1:10 to 2:1; Elizabeth, Luke 1:24 ff.; and
Mary, Luke 1:46 to 2:19.   •

Even Hagar, Genesis 16:4–13, who was no doubt a pagan before
her association with Abraham and Sarah, came to realize God's
loving protection over her and her unborn child, so that at the
child's birth she named him Ishmael, which means, "God hears."

In John 16:21 Jesus mentions the joy of a new mother at the
birth of her child, and contrasts it with the sober anxiety that pre-
cedes the birth. This contrast between the emotions of sorrow and
joy is a familiar one in Scripture, as in Esther 9:22; Nehemiah
8:10; Isaiah 35:10; Jeremiah 31:13, and so forth, and was not
new to the disciples to whom Jesus was speaking. In this parallel the
same words are used for each: *lupē—chaira* for the mother;
lupē—chaira for the disciples.

Jesus' understanding of the birth experience of a woman is evidenced further in the use of the word *thlipsis* to describe the labor. *Thlipsis,* or the verb forms, *thlibō, apōthlibō,* is sometimes translated symbolically as "oppression." But its literal meaning is to squeeze, compress, or press, as in Luke 8:45 and Mark 3:10, Phillips' translation:

> . . . the crowds are all around you and are *pressing* (**apōthlibo**) you on all sides.

> . . . all those . . . kept *pressing* (**thlibō**) forward to touch him.

The Latin translation of *thlipsis* in John 16:21 as *pressurae* gives conclusive evidence that this is the real meaning of the word. Although some might point out that Jesus was not speaking to his disciples in Greek, it can certainly be assumed that the Greek words John uses are as close a parallel to the original words as he can make them.

It is not strange that Jesus' awareness of a woman's birth experience is recorded, as such things were freely spoken of in the society in which He lived. An example of this is the statement of the woman who called out to him in public one day:

> Blessed is the womb that bare thee, and the paps which thou hast sucked! (Luke 11:27.)

Jesus did not rebuke her but told her of a far greater truth:

> Yes, but a far greater blessing to hear the word of God and obey it. (Luke 11:28, Phillips.)

The freedom with which such things were acknowledged is pointed out in a description of the social customs of that day:

> For the poor inhabitants of Jerusalem's crowded slums . . . the newly married couple had to spend their first nuptial night in the same room with the other members of the family. . . . In Galilee, this custom did not prevail and the bridal pair were allowed full privacy on the wedding night. The exhibition of delicacy on the part of the Galileans is especially remarkable

because in general they were far less modest and refined than the Judeans.[6]

CHUL, YALAD, AND RELATED WORDS

The correct meaning of the words *chul* and *yalad* has already been discussed at length in Chapter 10. It should be noted that *chul* has other apparent meanings when it is not used in reference to childbirth. In addition to this primary meaning of creating, or bringing forth, it can also be translated as "patience," as in Psalm 37:7:

Rest in the Lord, and *wait patiently* (**chul**) for him.

And it can also mean "whirl," which is probably its meaning in Judges 21:21, 23, where it is translated as "dance":

Behold, if the daughters of Shiloh come out to *dance* (**chul**) in dances, then come ye out of the vineyards, and catch you every man his wife. . . . And the children of Benjamin . . . took them wives . . . of them that *danced* (**chul**).

The parallelism of *chul-yalad* in reference to birth or creating is found too often to be disregarded. There are examples of it in the Pentateuch, in the Wisdom Literature, and in the Prophets. A few examples will illustrate this:

Knowest thou the time when the wild goats of the rock *bring forth* (**yalad**); Or canst thou mark when the hinds do *calve* (**chul**). (Job. 39:1.)

Art thou the first man that was *born* (**yalad**)? Or wast thou *made* (**chul**) before the hills? (Job 15:9.)

Before the mountains were *brought forth* (**yalad**), or ever thou hadst *formed* (**chul**) the earth and the world, even from everlasting to everlasting, thou art God. (Ps. 90:2.)

Before she was in *labor* (**chul**) she *gave birth* (**yalad**); . . . Shall a land be *born* (**chul**) in one day? Shall a nation be *brought forth* (**yalad**) in one moment? (Isa. 66:7, 8, RSV.)

To be consistent, verses like Isaiah 26:18 should be translated in this manner also, where the Authorized Version says "we have been in *pain* (**chul**)":

> We have been with child, we have been in *labor* (**chul**), we have as it were *brought forth* (**yalad**) wind. . . .

The three New Testament Greek words used of childbirth, *tiktō*, *gennaō*, and *ōdinō*, are also interchangeable and do not mean "pain." In the Septuagint, any one of the three is used to translate either *chul* or *yalad*. For example, *yalad* is translated as *ōdinō* in Isaiah 26:17; as *tiktō* in Isaiah 54:1; and as *gennaō* in Isaiah 26:18.

There are six additional Biblical words describing childbirth that remain to be discussed—one in the New Testament, and five in the Old Testament.

The New Testament word is *basanidzō*, which describes the efforts of the woman in the apocalyptic passage of Revelation 12:2, in giving birth. *Basanidzō* does not mean "pained to be delivered," as the passive phrase in the Authorized Version indicates; it means she was "straining with all her might" to give birth. Reverend J. B. Phillips illustrates this use of *basanidzō* in his translation of Mark 6:48: "He saw them *straining* (**basanidzō**) at the oars."

There is another verse in the New Testament where the Authorized Version adds the word "pain," although it does not appear in the Greek. This is in Romans 8:22, where the Greek says simply:

> The whole creation groans *in labor together* (**sunōdinō**) until now.

The five remaining Old Testament words used in connection with childbirth are *tsir, chaval, qashah, yaphach,* and *tsarah.*

1. *Tsir* is sometimes translated "hinges":

> As the door turneth upon his *hinges* (**tsir**) . . . (Prov. 26:14.)

Tsir is used of childbirth only once—in I Samuel 4:19, where the woman is said to crouch, or bend down, because her *tsir* had come upon her. *Tsir* is translated as "pains" in this verse, but we know this cannot be correct because Eli's daughter-in-law, absorbed with her grief, ignored the birth processes of her body and did not even realize when her child had been born until her attendants brought the fact to her attention.

It is possible that *tsir* refers here to the "hinges," or joints of the body as she crouches to give birth, but it is more likely that it refers to the opening of the door of the womb and the vulva. In the Talmud there are references to parts of the body in allegorical form that illustrate this: "In the Talmud the uterus is called the sleeping chamber, the cervix is the porch, the vagina the outer house, the clitoris the key, *the labia the hinges*, and the 'seed vessels' the store-room." (Italics added.)[7]

Tsir is used twice in Isaiah as a comparison to a woman giving birth. In Isaiah 13:8 it refers to the King of Babylon, and in Isaiah 21:3, to the prophet himself. In these two instances it probably refers to the "hinges" of the body as it assumes a crouching posture similar to "a woman giving birth."

2. *Chaval* is translated "cords, bands, bounds," over fifty times, and when used as a medical term is said to refer to muscles or nerves in action, as in a birth contraction. It is sometimes translated "pangs," but this English word is obsolete today, so "birth contraction" would be a more accurate translation. Sometimes *chaval* is translated simply "brought forth," as in Song of Solomon 8:5, which is also a poetic reference to a birth taking place in the out-of-doors:

> I raised thee up under the apple tree: there thy mother *brought thee forth* (**chaval**); there she *brought thee forth* (**chaval**) that bare thee.

3. *Qashah* is one of the three words used of childbirth in the Old Testament which implies an unhappy experience. *Qashah*, meaning "hard, difficult, fierce," is used of a birth only once, and

describes Rachel's difficult, abnormal delivery of Benjamin in Genesis 35:16, 17, where it is translated as "hard labor." In the Mishnah, the phrase "hard labor" is used of an animal who has difficulty in giving birth. Out of kindness, the attendant is instructed to destroy the offspring, and remove it limb by limb to save the life of the mother animal and to prevent her suffering. The Talmud applies this same principle to a mother who cannot give birth normally.

The two remaining words occur only in the Book of Jeremiah in connection with childbirth. It must be remembered that Jeremiah was a prophet among the indolent members of a court society, whose women would be likely to have more tiring labors than the peasant women of the same period. Therefore, these references in Jeremiah cannot be taken to mean that the same conditions applied throughout Old Testament times, or even to women generally in Jeremiah's day. Furthermore, Jeremiah prohesied in a time of national disaster, when fear and apprehension were prevalent, especially at court. It has already been demonstrated how fear creates physical tension, which in turn creates pain. Thus we would expect these women to have more difficulty in their labors.

The two words Jeremiah uses do not mean "pain," but they do refer to conditions that would cause unhappiness and imply suffering. These two words are *yaphach*, and *tsarah*.

4. *Yaphach*, meaning "gasping," "out of breath," or "to breathe oneself out," is used of a woman in labor only once in the Bible, in Jeremiah 4:31. This verse describes her condition as one of complete exhaustion, as she labors to deliver her firstborn child. She becomes so weak with exhaustion that she cannot even close her hands around a support any longer to help herself in bearing down.

5. *Tsarah*, used figuratively, is commonly translated "distress," but it can also convey the idea of constriction, narrowness, or "straits," as in the following passages:

> . . . the place where we dwell is too *strait* (**tsarah**) for us. (II Kings 6:1.)

> . . . the place is too *strait* (**tsarah**) for me, give place to me that I may dwell. (Isa. 49:20.)

> The angel of the Lord went further, and stood in a *narrow* (**tsarah**) place. (Num. 22:26.)

> For the bed is shorter than that a man can stretch himself on it: and the covering *narrower* (**tsarah**) than that he can wrap himself in it. (Isa. 28:20.)

Tsarah is used in verses that contain a comparison to labor six times in Jeremiah. Three of these times it refers to the woman: (a) 4:31 (see the discussion of *yaphach*, above); (b) 48:41, which also has the element of being surprised, and seems to imply that the woman is afraid; and (c) 49:22, which also implies the presence of fear. Whether *tsarah* refers to the "constriction" of a contraction in these three verses, or to an emotional "distress," is not too important, since in each case a distressing situation is implied by the context.

In the three other places where Jeremiah uses *tsarah* there is reference to the approaching confinement of captivity—the nation will be "in a bind." Here again, *tsarah* may have a double meaning and imply distress as well as captivity. In these three passages it is not clear whether the phrase in which *tsarah* appears is a part of the comparison to a "woman in labor" or not. The word is applied to (a) the inhabitants of Zion, 6:24; (b) Damascus, 49:24; and (c) the King of Babylon, 50:43.

THE SEPTUAGINT AND ENGLISH TRANSLATIONS

It is worthy of note that the simile, "as a woman giving birth," which appears fifteen times in our English translations of the Old Testament, appears only nine times in the Septuagint. This simile occurs only once in the Old Testament outside of the prophetical literature, and this is in Psalm 48:6, where it tells of the kings "*laboring* (**chul**) as a woman *giving birth* (**yalad**)." This is a comparison of the effort syndrome in rowing to the effort syndrome of giving birth. The kings are rowing with all their might to escape the impending destruction from God, symbolized by the "east wind." The picture is like that of Mark 6:48 (Phillips) where the disciples are "straining at the oars."

But this simile does not appear in the Septuagint! The entire passage is a different one, and verses 4–7 read as follows:

> My mouth shall speak wisdom,
> And the meditation of my heart knowledge.
> I shall incline my ear to a parable,
> I shall open my defense with the harp.
> Why do I fear in the evil day?
> The lawlessness of my foot shall surround me.

The simile "as a woman giving birth" is also missing from the Septuagint in Jeremiah 30:6; 48:41; 49:22, 24; and 50:43. Of the nine times it does appear, five times either a phrase is left out or it is interpreted differently from our English translations.

1. In Isaiah 13:8 the phrase "and they shall be afraid" is missing, and the phrase translated into English as "*pangs* (**tsir**) and *sorrows* (**chaval**) shall take hold on them" reads:

> . . . the aged ones will be thrown into a tumult (*kai tarax-thēsontai hoi presbeis*).

2. In Isaiah 21:3 the word translated *pain* (**chul**) is translated *ekluō*, which means "to give out, become weak, loosen, or become weary." In medicine, when *ekluō* is used in connection with the word for "loins," as it is here, it is a term used for involuntary defecation —a releasing of the contents of the bowel, as a mother releases her child from the birth canal. In this same verse, the Septuagint omits the phrase, "*pangs* (**tsir**) have taken hold on me" (that is, on the prophet himself).

3. In Isaiah 42:14, rather than having the Lord say ". . . now will I *cry* (**paah**) like a *travailing* (**yalad**) woman," as the Authorized Version reads, the Septuagint authors render this verse as:

> I have been as *patient* (**katereō**) as a woman *giving birth* (**tiktō**).

The Hebrew word *paah* then, probably refers in this verse to the groan of effort of the Lord, like the groan of a woman in labor—a groan that is a normal part of the effort syndrome in even the most painless birth. In the Brown, Driver, Briggs *Lexicon*, this phrase is explained as meaning that "the Lord [is] straining himself to deliver Israel."[8]

In Isaiah 26:17, where the woman *crieth out* (**zaaq**) in labor, this same explanation might apply. In the Seputagint *zaaq* is translated as *ekkradzō* in this verse, and means "to call out, cry, or shout." *Kradzō* is even used in classical writings sometimes to describe the noise frogs make!

4. In Jeremiah 4:31 the Septuagint uses *stenagmos* ("groan") to translate the Hebrew word *tsarah*, thus relating the word to the effort of labor.

5. The garbled meaning of Micah 4:9, 10, as it is translated into English, is a vivid contrast to its apparent meaning as it appears in the Septuagint. In the RSV these verses read:

> Now why do you cry aloud?
>   Is there no king in you?
> Has your counselor perished
>   that *pangs* (**chul**) have seized you
>   like a woman in *travail* (**yalad**)?
> *Writhe* (**chul**) and groan, O daughter of Zion
>   like a woman in *travail* (**yalad**);
>   for now you shall go forth from the city. . . .
>   you shall go to Babylon.
> There you shall be rescued,
>   there the Lord will redeem you
>   from the hand of your enemies.

The really ironic thing about this mistranslation is that it occurs right in the *center* of Micah's message of comfort to his people, which begins at the opening of the fourth chapter and leads up to the promise of the Messiah in Chapter 5. In other words, our translators would have us believe that Micah is telling the people that they are going to "writhe" in "pangs" like a woman in labor, because God has graciously promised to rescue them from the enemy.

Translators have inserted concepts of suffering in other passages of comfort and blessing that refer to childbirth, as in Isaiah 54:1–4; 66:7–9; Jeremiah 31:8, etc. Their doing this reminds one of Job's comment to his friends in Job 16:2: "Miserable comforters are ye all!"

What Micah is saying in 4:9, 10 in comforting Judah is that they should not continue to weep as if there were no hope. He has already given them the glad news that "the mountain of the house of the Lord shall be established" (verse 1). "Is there no king in you?" he asks gently. "Has your counselor perished, that you labor like a woman giving birth?"

Micah's comparison here brings to mind Dr. Dick-Read's picture of the "hard-working woman employing the effort syndrome, which made her appear distressed." Micah encourages Judah to "groan and labor, like a woman giving birth . . . for you will be delivered."

The Septuagint also shows that Micah is here telling the "daughter of Zion" to take courage, as one might encourage a woman nearing delivery:

> And now why have you known evils? Was there not a king for you? Or did your counsel perish that labor as of one who gives birth has taken hold of you?
>
> Be in labor, but be courageous and draw near, daughter of Zion, as one who gives birth. Because now you will go out of a city and live in the field and you will go to Babylon. From there He will save you and from there the Lord your God will redeem you out of the hands of your enemies.

In the remaining four passages in the Septuagint that contain the simile "as a woman giving birth" (Isaiah 26:17; Jeremiah 6:24; 13:19; 22:23), the words *tiktō*, *gennaō*, or *odinō* are used where the English erroneously translates the Hebrew as "travail," "pain," or "pangs."

In order to understand how English renderings can differ so much from the Septuagint, one must realize that our English and European translations of the Old Testament are based primarily on the Hebrew Masoretic text, of which the earliest extant manuscript dates back only to A.D. 895. To what extent the Masoretic text is corrupt in places where it differs from the Septuagint is a problem that linguistic scholars struggle to determine. Regardless of their decisions, the importance of the Septuagint, with its happier renderings of childbirth passages, can hardly be overestimated: *It was the only Old Testament widely used by the early Church throughout the Greek-speaking world until the Latin Vulgate appeared in the fourth and fifth centuries* A.D.

Many New Testament quotations from the Old Testament were taken by the New Testament writers word for word from the Septuagint. And although the Septuagint was thoroughly Jewish in origin, it became so identified with the Christian Church that the Jews finally sponsored another Greek translation of their own by a Jew named Aquila.

By the time the Latin Vulgate replaced the Septuagint in the Church, a change in the attitude of many Christian writers, including Jerome, toward a woman's sexual functions as wife and childbearer was already well under way.

However, a negative attitude toward women was still evident at the time the Authorized Version was translated in A.D. 1611, so that many mistranslations of childbirth words occurred. But the really surprising thing is that it is the translators of some of the newer revisions of the last half century who have been the chief offenders in this regard. In their attempts to break away from awkward literal translating and use familiar English words, they have unwittingly "read into" the text the concept of childbirth pain in many places where it is not in the original languages, nor even in the Authorized Version. This is understandable because of the emphasis on the inevitability of pain in childbirth in our culture, and its seeming confirmation by the shocking sufferings in childbirth of the eighteenth and nineteenth centuries.

As a matter of fact, many of us are guilty of careless "reading into" the text our own concepts of childbirth pain. In I Thessalonians 5:3, for example, how many people have thought that Paul was comparing the terrifying experience of destruction to the "terrifying" experience of giving birth?

> For when they shall say, Peace and safety; then sudden destruction cometh upon them, as travail upon a woman with child; and they shall not escape.

In interpreting a verse like this it is important to determine just what the points of comparison are. In this verse there are two:

1. The *time* of destruction—it comes when it is unexpected, as labor may begin before the mother is prepared. It's "ready or not, here I come!" when a child is ready to be born.

2. The *certainty* of destruction—as certain as that a pregnant woman must some day give birth to a child. She cannot change her mind, or even put it off to some more convenient time.

THE TALMUD AND CHURCH INTERPRETATIONS

The Jewish emphasis upon the blessings of marriage and parenthood has already been mentioned. This emphasis is stressed in the Talmud:

> An entire section of the Talmud is devoted to "The Obligation to marry and to propagate the race." To refuse to do so is tantamount to bloodshed and to expelling the Divine Presence from Israel.[9]

Of the fifty references to Eve listed in the index of the Soncino edition of the Talmud, there is only one passage that mentions any "curse" of Eve. This "curse" is interpreted as being in ten parts, embracing the whole area of a woman's life. The "pain" of childbirth is not mentioned, and the phrase, "in *etsev* shalt thou bring forth children" is dismissed with the statement, "to be understood in its literal meaning."

The "curse" of Adam is paired with Eve's and is divided into ten parts also. Jewish literature does not single out Eve as bearing a special punishment but mentions her side by side with Adam's. In fact, Rabbi Johanan, one of the most prominent of the early rabbis, says that a man's punishment was "twice as great." This is certainly different from the doctrine of the Church these last centuries. In another place in the Talmud we read of Eve:

> Because she was the mother of all living she was given (to her husband) to live, but not to suffer pain.[10]

Rabbi Jakobovits quotes the Talmud as saying that a woman "is not bound to torment herself on account of her submission to her husband," and that "one need not destroy oneself in order to populate the world."[11]

Among the early Jewish writings outside the Talmud, a reference is found to the "sentence" to which Eve was subjected. In this explanation (c. A.D. 300) of Eve's sentence found in the Tosephta of Rabbi Nathan, the *birth* of a child is not included at all!

> As Adam was laid under three sentences, likewise was it with Eve. . . . The first few days of menstruation are painful. So also are the first few moments of sexual intercourse with a man. Also, when a woman becomes pregnant, her face loses its beauty and becomes yellow the first three months.

Since the Talmud does not condemn women to suffering, the objections raised by the Church to the use of anesthetics in labor are not paralleled in Jewish thought.

> The question about the prohibition of painless birth in view of Gen. III, 16 is never found in the *Responsa*. As far back as the time of the Renaissance an Italian Rabbi—R. Obadiah Sforno (1475–1550)—did not interpret the Hebrew word "teldi" (thou shalt bring forth) literally. According to him the meaning of the word "teldi" is: "thou shalt bring up," *i.e.,* thou shalt bring up thy children in pain more than any other creature has to endure in bringing up its offspring. Prohibition of analgesics would contradict Jewish ideology, according to which the ways of the *Torah* "are of pleasantness, and all her paths are peace." (Prov. III, 17.)[12]

The Jewish attitude toward the Genesis passage gives us insight into other references to childbirth in the Bible. It is a clue to Paul's meaning when he uses the word *teknogonia* ("childbearing") in I Timothy 2:15. Although Paul became a Christian, he also calls himself "an Hebrew of the Hebrews" (Philippians 3:5), and evidences of his Hebrew background are seen here. Some have interpreted *teknogonia* as a reference to the "curse of Eve," by which they mean that a woman who lives a godly, Christian life will be protected from pain or death during childbirth and have an easy delivery. Such an interpretation by Christians was sharply questioned even a century ago, when the outcry by the Church against any relief of pain in childbirth was at its height:

> [One scholar] represents the *teknogonia* as that in which the curse finds its operation (an extravagant statement to begin with, since *death* was plainly set forth as for both man and woman the proper embodiment of the curse), then, that she was to be exempted from this curse in its worst and heaviest effects (of which, however, nothing is said in the original word), and that besides, she should be saved *through*—that is, passing through the curse of her child-bearing trials—saved, notwithstanding the danger and distress connected with these! Surely a most unnatural and forced explanation, and ending in a very lame and impotent conclusion![13]

It is more consistent with the context of this passage to translate *teknogonia* as "motherhood," as the translators of the New English Bible have done. E. J. Goodspeed, in his translation of the New Testament, also translates this word as "motherhood." Such a translation is in keeping with the similar injunction to women given by Paul in Titus 2:3 (New English Bible):

> The older women . . . must set a high standard, and school the younger women to be loving wives and mothers, temperate, chaste, and kind, busy at home, respecting the authority of their own husbands.

Protestant theologians are not the only ones who have come to the conclusion that such passages are references to "motherhood" rather than to "childbirth." Pope Pius XII, in an address on natural childbirth in 1956, outlined the official Catholic position. He says in part:

> . . . God did not wish to forbid and did not forbid men to seek after and make use of all the riches of creation; to make progress

step by step in culture; to make life in this world more bearable
and better; to lighten the burden of work and fatigue, pain,
sickness and death, in a word to subdue the earth (Genesis, i,
28). . . . God did not wish to forbid—nor did he forbid—
mothers to make use of means which render childbirth easier and
less painful. One must not seek subterfuges for the words of
sacred scripture: They remain true in the sense intended and expressed by the Creator, namely: motherhood will give the mother
much suffering to bear.[14]

As has been noted before, the attitude toward motherhood in New
Testament and early Church days was similar to that of the Jews of
the same period. This attitude is little changed today. Rabbi Jakobovits sums up the difference between Jewish and Christian attitudes toward childbirth during some of the intervening centuries by
comparing their respective attitudes toward suffering in general:

> There is no trace in rabbinic law of the Christian concept in
> which "Pathos became Ethos; suffering was a sign of grace, not
> to be evaded but sought." It is true, the moral codes of the Church
> also modified many of its principles for the sake of mitigating
> pain. . . . But in general, Christianity is distinctly more panegyrical
> in its commendation of physical suffering than is Judaism.[15]

Although excesses such as flagellation are no longer countenanced
by the Church, some Christians still believe that all suffering is the
result of sin and that patient bearing of pain is a sign of repentance
and humility. But the Reverend J. S. Stewart shows how all suffering
cannot be attributed to sin, and that many of the tragedies in life are
due to the inexorability of the laws which govern the universe, and
yet that it is the very rigidity of these laws upon which life depends:

> Take even grim facts like earthquakes and volcanoes. It is
> hard to discover any trace of beneficence there. But the fact is
> that the very forces which occasionally produce these devastating
> outbursts are the same forces which, working continually beneath
> the earth's surface, make and keep this planet habitable for the
> sons of men. You cannot have all the assets of life, and refuse
> its liabilities.[16]

So it is that in the normal process of childbirth there are factors, such as disproportion of the baby's head in relation to the mother's pelvis, or muscular resistance to the birth, which may give rise to pain. But that such pain is the result of Eve's sin is a concept that cannot be considered an adequate Christian explanation.

But what if Genesis 3:16 could be interpreted as meaning that physical pain in childbirth is the judgment for sin; what if the passages in the prophets could be interpreted as meaning that all women in Bible history writhed in pain in childbirth, and that all births everywhere since the beginning of time have been agony. Would this "prove" that natural childbirth is not scriptural? Not at all. The basic principles of God's Holy Word, which reveal God as a perfect and loving Creator, also reveal that it is His desire that the sufferings of this present world be alleviated, and that all mankind, through Christ, be brought into physical and spiritual harmony with their Maker. With these principles the philosophy of natural childbirth is in harmony.

Notes

1. Rabbi Samson Raphael Hirsch, *The Pentateuch* (London: Isaac Levy, 1959), Vol. I, p. 83.
2. *Ibid.,* p. 85.
3. Flavius Josephus, *Jewish Antiquities*, trans. Thackeray, Loeb Classical Library (London: Heinemann, 1889), Book I, p. 83.
4. Irenaeus, "Irenaeus Against Heresies," Book III, Chap. XXIII, in *The Ante-Nicene Fathers* (Grand Rapids, Mich.: Eerdmans, 1951).
5. George Foot Moore, *Judaism* (Cambridge: Harvard University Press, 1950), Vol. I, p. 445.
6. Louis Finkelstein, *The Pharisees* (Philadelphia: Jewish Publication Society of America, 1946), p. 47.
7. H. J. Zimmels, *Magicians, Theologians and Doctors* (London: Goldston, 1952), p. 16.
8. Brown, Driver, Briggs, *A Hebrew and English Lexicon of the Old Testament* (London: Oxford, 1907).
9. Rabbi Immanuel Jakobovits, *Jewish Medical Ethics* (New York: Philosophical Library, 1959), p. 154.

10. The Talmud, Kheth, I, 364.
11. Jakobovits, *Jewish Medical Ethics,* p. 165.
12. Zimmels, *Magicians, Theologians and Doctors,* p. 7.
13. Patrick Fairbairn, *The Pastoral Epistles* (Edinburgh: T. and T. Clark, 1874).
14. "Text of Address by Pope Pius XII on the Science and Morality of Natural Childbirth," printed in the *New York Times,* January 9, 1956, from the official Vatican translation of Pope Pius' address in French on January 8.
15. Jakobovits, *Jewish Medical Ethics.*
16. J. S. Stewart, *The Strong Name* (Edinburgh: T. and T. Clark, 1941), pp. 137, 138.

Chapter 19

Contemporary Obstetric Practices

INTRODUCTION

It is not surprising, when one realizes the historical background of modern obstetrics, that certain basic misunderstandings persist. One can see how knowledge that the staggering death rate from puerperal fever was caused by filthy conditions led to such an emphasis on sterile, aseptic deliveries that human relationships became sterile as well. Because of the emphasis on asepsis, the emotional needs of the three human beings involved in the birth are overlooked.

Nor is it difficult to see how the terrible suffering and deaths in childbed of the centuries preceding ours have led to overemphasis on the necessity of anesthetic relief in humane attempts to prevent such suffering.

Also, a realization of some of the erroneous religious concepts that have influenced our American and European cultures helps us to appreciate why our societies, including the medical profession, have been so slow in accepting a more positive approach to childbirth.

This chapter reveals some of the painful results of the inadequate concepts of childbirth that we have inherited. These facts are not pleasant to relate, and the reader must realize that they are accusations against a *philosophy,* and the consequent *methods* of modern obstetrics, not accusations against medical personnel or their motives. Doctors, too, are victims of our negative concepts of childbirth. They have suffered when their patients suffered, and if at times they have seemed indifferent to a woman's pain it is because they felt they had to keep a purely objective and scientific attitude toward their patients to function efficiently as physicians. But the more humane ones feel a genuine sympathy for the pain during childbirth that they witness day after day.

INADEQUACIES

1. *An inadequate philosophy is reflected in inadequate training in obstetrics for medical personnel.* The prevalence of medieval and Victorian concepts of childbirth pain among medical personnel in this second half of the twentieth century is a reflection of their inadequate training in philosophy and the humanities. Because of this lack, some of them are unable to comprehend that pain in a typical birth might have a logical, rational explanation. Their concept is that pain during labor and during the delivery is *normal* rather than symptomatic of abnormal conditions. In no other function of the healthy human body is "pain" regarded as a normal accompaniment.

It is not surprising to find this concept of pain in a book written by a doctor in 1929:

> The pains accompany the intermittent contractions of the muscle of the uterus as it attempts to expel its contents, and arise from this contraction . . . the time between them decreases as the labor progresses and their intensity increases. The most severe pain, the agony of childbirth, comes after the child's head has passed from the uterus and while it is propelled through the vagina. The passage is stretched and sometimes torn; the pain is often extremely severe.[1]

It *is* most surprising to find this concept still expressed in a recent book by a doctor.

> The reality of pain during labor and delivery is so deeply engraved in our own as well as in practically every other culture that it is indeed an intrepid soul who would deny its existence. . . .

It is indeed difficult to believe that pain is not one of the primary components of the ordinary process of parturition under any circumstances. . . . The sublimation of pain may be one of the explanations of the apparent ability of some women to go through labor and delivery *presumably* without pain.[2]

Because the concept of pain as a normal accompaniment of labor and birth is so deeply embedded in the minds of many doctors, they have dismissed as "irrational" the statements and evidences from women who have experienced happy childbirths. In books and articles they have written that these mothers show evidence of "hysteria" or that they are masochistic and have simply "sublimated" pain as pleasure. Or they insist that these mothers "hypnotized" themselves. When many have tried to explain that childbirth was not only a profoundly moving emotional experience but also a physical pleasure akin to orgasm, the doctors are convinced that such mothers are unbalanced. One doctor wrote:

> The author actually heard one patient who had been well-conditioned psychologically for parturition compare the fulfillment and satisfaction of the moment of the birth of the child to that of the sensation of a sexual orgasm! . . . One would also be interested in knowing a little more about the patient's innate emotional stability.[3]

Because of an inadequate philosophy concerning childbirth, the teaching of obstetrics in medical schools is often concerned primarily with the problem of abnormal obstetrics. Consequently, every normal labor as well is considered by some doctors as an "obstetric case" and submitted to the same rigid routine. Dr. Herbert Ratner, director of the Department of Public Health in Oak Park, Illinois, illustrates this clearly:

> . . . Take, say, the obstetrical specialist, a key specialist who cuts into the heart of family practice. For his own self-justification he stops thinking of pregnancy as a normal physiological condition and permits himself to believe that it is a pathological condition requiring specialized attention. It was a modern obstetrician who defined pregnancy as a nine-month disease. . . . To think of preg-

nancy as a disease with all the implications this has for the mother undergoing the experience . . . contributes nothing of value to the mental health of the family unit. This is especially so when the concept of pregnancy as a disease is matched by the specialist's concept of a delivery appropriate to the occasion: routine forceps, anesthesia, and episiotomies with the attendant stuporousness, emesis basins, and sore bottoms. The unnatural delivery, with only short-term clinical experience behind it, displaces natural delivery, the product of thousands of years of evolutionary experience which also had the virtue of preserving the mother for the moment of joy inherent in the birth of a baby.[4]

Dr. Ratner correctly points out that this unfortunate approach has arisen partly because of a failure to develop a *philosophy* concerning the practice of medicine. He suggests that medicine should be considered as an "art" rather than a "science" and that medical students should be challenged as "humanitarians, not as technologists." This is particularly important for the student of obstetrics.

2. *Inadequate prenatal care and training for expectant parents, with resultant inadequate rapport between childbearing women and their doctors.*

It has been estimated that in the United States alone there are as many as 100,000 women who deliver their babies every year without having any prenatal care. Something must be done to help women learn the importance of medical supervision during pregnancy and childbirth. And someone must make provision for this care, which is being done in countries with socialized medicine.

Many women go to the doctor during pregnancy. But after the health examination of the first office visit, most of them simply go through the following routine each successive time: they are weighed, have their urine tested, their blood pressure taken, and their abdomen palpated. Of course, these procedures are essential, but they are not explained to the women so that they know why they are being done. Then, after a peremptory "Any questions?" they are told when to return and summarily dismissed. This represents the sum total of their training for one of the most important experiences of their whole lives.

Most doctors ask an expectant mother if she has any questions. But this is not sufficient. One young woman complained to me that the doctor asking this didn't help her at all. "My whole mind is one big question," she said. "I don't know enough to ask an intelligent question, and yet there is so much I want to know." This girl was a college graduate. She showed me her physiology textbook with its description and diagrams of the process of birth. And still she said that her mind was "one big question."

Fortunately, prenatal classes are springing up all over the world. Some of these classes are helpful. Some are a waste of time. There are two basic things a young woman wants to know when she attends a prenatal class. She wants to know, "What is going to happen to *me?*" and "How can I help *myself* when the time comes?" This introspective self-interest is a normal reaction to pregnancy. She is less interested in the physiology of birth, style shows, and how to care for the baby, although these are helpful, too.

Evidence is mounting which shows that adequate prenatal education is an essential component of good maternity care. Dr. M. Edward Davis of the University of Chicago School of Medicine writes:

> Is parent education effective? Experiences at Chicago Lying-In ... have convinced me that it is the most important part of modern pre-natal care. It has resulted in a marked decrease in the incidence of prolonged labor, a reduction in the need for analgesia, and fewer complicated deliveries.[5]

3. *Inadequate relief from pain during childbirth, in spite of the employment of analgesics and anesthetics beyond the limits of safety.*

It is a common misconception that the natural childbirth patient is a "stoic," while the orthodox obstetric patient is relieved of her pain by means of drugs. Quite the opposite is true. The natural childbirth patient, because she knows how to prevent pain from occurring by relaxation and proper breathing, does not suffer, while the untrained orthodox patient, because she is tense, does feel severe pain even under sedation. The oversedated mother, whose child may be adversely affected, suffers pain and tosses in a drunken stupor. If she is completely unconscious during this time she may not remember the pain afterward, but more often she does remember some unhappy portions of her experience. Because the drugs cause one to lose all self-control, what one does remember often assumes an embarrassing, nightmarish quality. Dr. Thom explains this aspect of the use of drugs:

> In the use of these amnesic drugs I would add for the sake of the uninformed that their side effects sometimes produce such excitation that for protection patients have to be put in restraint-type beds and other devices used reminiscent of a medieval madhouse.[6]

When there is muscular tension, the pain during labor feels very similar to menstrual cramps when menstruation is delayed. Of course, during labor this pain is distributed over a larger area. In painful menstruation, the pain does not seem to be so much in the tiny uterus itself, as in the tense, aching, congested muscles that surround it. This throbbing pain spreads throughout the lower abdomen, across the lower back, throughout the tissues of the pelvic area, and even down into the thighs. It can become so severe that one can hardly stand or sit up straight. The same thing happens in labor, and the pain of contractions is felt primarily in all the tissues that *surround* the uterus, rather than in the uterus itself. When the muscles of these areas are consciously relaxed, this pain miraculously disappears, and the woman feels only the uterus contracted firmly, but with no more unpleasantness than a contracted bicep in her arm.

During my teen years I frequently suffered severe cramps from delayed menstruation. Finally I discovered, by trial and error, that if I went to bed and became warm enough to *relax* all the muscles in the abdominal and pelvic area of my body and fall into a quiet sleep, I would awaken an hour or two later to find the pain gone and the menstrual flow well established. I could then get up and go about my regular duties with no further discomfort. The pain had been caused by unconscious muscular tension, which had inhibited menstruation. Years later, when I first read of the relationship of muscle tension to pain in labor, the importance of relaxing at this time immediately made good sense to me.

If a natural childbirth patient has difficulty relaxing, a mild sedative may be given. But many women, trained for natural childbirth, have complained that their attendants have given them too large a dose so that they have lost *conscious muscular control* of relaxation. Consequently, they reacted to the drugs in the usual irrational, painful way, unable to relax.

It can no longer be denied that natural childbirth shortens labor and lessens discomfort to the point where little or no sedation is needed. Of the more than two thousand women who had their babies in this manner in the joint Maternity Center Association–Yale project, the following report was given:

> In 34 per cent of 257 [primiparas] the first stage was 6 hours or less. In 63 per cent it was 10 hours or less. . . . Our own ex-experience has convinced us that under our present regime we have a greatly lessened number of depressed infants at birth, a decrease in the length of labors, fewer operative deliveries, less blood loss, smoother convalescence, and finally, happier mothers.[7]

In natural childbirth, sedation (usually Demerol) is given according to individual needs and desires, rather than as a routine at a given point in a woman's labor. Very often sedation is not needed at all. On occasions when it may be necessary, the amount given is varied according to individual need. Dr. William Rashbaum emphasized this recently when he said that the sedation—if needed at all, might be

> . . . twenty-five milligrams with this patient and perhaps 125 with another patient. This is the art of medicine and also the advantage of individual medical attention.[8]

4. *Inadequate consideration for the parturient woman's simple comfort.*

One of the most disliked procedures of orthodox obstetrics is the enema. Some doctors are finally becoming aware of this and are experimenting with less distressing ways of obtaining a clean field for delivery. In Russia the enema is given only if it is needed. In France a mother following the psychoprophylactic method of natural childbirth gives herself an enema before leaving home. At the International Childbirth Education Association convention in June 1962, in Seattle, Washington, some doctors reported that they did not have their patients shaved at all and that the enema was given only if needed. In the *American Journal of Obstetrics and Gynecology,* September 15, 1962, an article written by a doctor, "The Enema—Is It Necessary?" suggests that one alternative is the use of a simple suppository.

> The physician who is not present during the administration of the enema is usually unaware of the patient's discomfort and even embarrassment during this procedure. Labor and delivery should be as pleasant and physiologic as possible, yet the patient's admission usually starts with a most displeasing experience. . . . The soapsuds enema has disadvantages in addition to the patient's discomfort. It is irritating to the mucosa. Trauma, including perforation of the rectum, may be caused by the enema tube, and enema fluid may contaminate the small bowel. . . . Side effects caused by general discomfort, mild or marked cramps, and rectal irritation amounted to 84.8 per cent in the enema group [of the 1,159 patients tested] compared to 1.5 per cent for the bisacodyl [suppository] patients.[9]

A second intensely disliked experience is the irritated soreness of perineal tissue after childbirth, due to an episiotomy and repair. New mothers in maternity wards sometimes disrespectfully refer to their painful attempts at walking while this soreness persists as "the hemorrhoid shuffle." The sore area is soaked in sitz baths, heated with lamps, plastered with salves in attempts to hasten the healing and ease the discomfort. The orthodox physician performs an episiotomy nearly 100 per cent of the time.

There is growing evidence that the episiotomy is not really necessary. It has been pointed out that a muscle in good condition has a stretch ratio of 8 to 1, so that when a mother has practiced vaginal contractions during pregnancy, she is able to contract or relax these muscles at will during birth. By relaxing them, she keeps them from offering resistance to the birth of the child, so that her labor is shortened and her tissues do not tear. However, episiotomies may still be necessary in some instances, as in the birth of a premature child, when the tissues have not been fully softened by hormones in preparation for the birth.

Additional advantages of the vaginal exercise listed by doctors are: better control over leaking of urine in later pregnancy; quicker healing of stitches following birth if an episiotomy had to be performed; restored vaginal resiliency soon after childbirth, so that the pleasure of intercourse is increased for both husband and wife; and a decreased need for surgery on cystoceles and rectoceles due to flabby vaginal walls in later life.

Dr. Arnold Kegel, gynecologist at the University of Southern California, has prepared a motion picture for professionals that demonstrates the advantages of this exercise.

Niles Newton graphically depicts the difference between an orthodox delivery, with episiotomy, and Dr. Dick-Read's procedure during the second stage of labor:

> When delivery seems imminent, the American woman is suddenly transported from her bed, pushed into a room with brilliant lights and medical instruments. She is then put on a special table that has equipment for tying her hands and feet, and her buttocks are adjusted so that she pushes her baby out into space, with no mattress to break its fall should the doctor fail to catch it. Labor is then quite usually artificially shortened by cutting the woman's perineum.
>
> In contrast to this, Read's patients are not routinely hauled into a frightening new environment just as the baby is about to emerge. Read advocates a much more leisurely second stage of labor. . . .[10]

As a result, Dr. Newton points out that 79 per cent of Dr. Dick-Read's primiparas were delivered without episiotomies and that they had intact perineums or just abrasions (first-degree tears requiring one or two stitches). And 96 per cent of his multiparas gave birth to their babies without incisions or tearing.

How many doctors can match his record?

The nurse-midwives of the Maternity Center Association can match it. Of the 4,988 mothers they delivered in homes, there was only one third-degree tear, and only twenty-two episiotomies were performed.

Most physicians justify their routinely cutting every woman by saying that if they don't, these women will be plagued with cystoceles and rectoceles in later life. This argument was effectively refuted by physicians who attended the International Childbirth Education Association (ICEA) convention in June 1962. One New Jersey physician reported that his patients of the preceding twelve years who had had adequate training and information and carefully controlled deliveries showed no tendency to prolapse as a result of a lack of episiotomies. Previously such prolapse had been frequent. A physician from Buffalo, New York, reported that he had taken over the practice of an elderly physician who had delivered his patients without medication or episiotomies and that the pelves of these women remained in excellent condition. Other physicians pointed out that rectoceles and cystoceles commonly occur in patients who *have* had episiotomies, so this is not an effective prevention. Dr. Morris Gold, of the Lynnwood Clinic in Lynnwood, Washington, describes in a personal communication how he preserves the perineum and why he believes it is necessary to do so:

> Many women, whether they openly express it or not, have a very real horror of having their perineums cut. Others feel that if while fully conscious and completing the second stage of delivery, they were to be advanced upon with hypodermic and scissors, it would spoil their moment of triumph. My patients expect me to preserve the perineum intact after delivery, if it is at all possible.
>
> My method, not at all new or original, is to deliver the baby slowly and carefully, while the mother pants, supporting the head off the pelvic floor. In this way 55% have no stitches at all, another 30% have a superficial laceration involving 1 or 2 stitches, 13% a second degree laceration. About 2% need an episiotomy when it is obvious that a tear is inevitable. All these are repaired with no tension on the stitches and we get almost no complaint of stitch pain. On later examination I find these women to have good muscle tone and pelvic support.
>
> On the question of saving the fetus the "pounding of the head upon the pelvic floor," I am aware of the theory of this "danger"

and the measures said to prevent it, supported by most obstetricians. However, it is hard to understand how a pair of forceps locked upon the fetal head with traction supplied by a strong adult, could do *less* damage than the maternal soft parts after the head has come through the bony pelvis. I have never seen convincing proof that this is so. And some wag has said that millions of doctors living and dead would never have thought of the perineum as something to be compared to a brick wall!

The conscientious physician gives his patient what she wants, only if it happens to be good for her. If I believed that I could prevent brain damage in children, or pelvic problems for my patients, I would of course do the episiotomy. However, like brain damage, the problem of prolapse is very complicated, involving many other factors in our culture: until there is a scientific study done which proves the episiotomy will prevent this pathological relaxation, I cannot deny my patients the ideal delivery and post partum comfort and mobility they hope for.

How do the Russians, with their great emphasis on science and physical vigor (all Russians are requested to do ten minutes of calisthenics daily, following instructions given over the radio by the government), help their women to avoid cystoceles and rectoceles? Certainly not by using routine episiotomies. The *Report of the Medical Exchange Mission to the USSR* relates that the incidence of episiotomies is only 9 to 11 per cent. All Russian women have prenatal classes available in which they are taught exercises in preparation for childbirth. Eighty-six per cent of these women participate in the classes, and of these, those who require medication for pain relief in labor vary from 8 to 14 per cent. No enema is given unless absolutely necessary. Forceps are used less than 2 per cent of the time. The incidence of Cesarean deliveries is 1 per cent. It is obvious that their system of preparing mothers for childbirth through education, relaxation, and exercises not only results in healthier, intact perineums but has many other benefits as well.

But while the enema and the episiotomy, used routinely in the United States for a woman in childbirth, are troublesome, there is one really cruel procedure in American obstetrics. This is the practice of strapping a woman down tightly flat on her back, often blindfolding her as well, during the second stage of labor. Of course, straps and protective eye coverings are necessary when a patient is unconscious under an anesthetic, but they have no justification whatever for a conscious, co-operative woman.

This American obstetric custom of strapping the laboring woman in an inflexible position is inexcusable. Her arms are pinned stiffly down alongside her body so that she cannot bend her elbows when pulling on the hand grips while bearing down. Her legs are pinned tightly in one rigid position (and *higher* than her head!), and her head is left flat on the hard delivery table, or, at best, is placed on a flat, skimpy pillow.

This customary lithotomy position makes labor difficult and exhausting, especially for the primipara. Many women have not realized that the severe backache and fatigue that troubled them in the days after their baby was born was due to their having abused their back muscles by arching their backs while pushing— the only way you *can* push when you are pinned flat on your back. Imagine trying to lift a weight from the ground, by arching your back and throwing your head back! Try it! Even a passive delivery in this position causes backache later, if one is pinned down in this way for any length of time.

Nurses always prop up patients to a semisitting position when they are brought the bedpans, if they are well enough, but how often is this same simple thoughtfulness expressed for the mother straining to deliver her child?

The use of this dorsal position for delivering a child was first popularized in the seventeenth century by Mauriceau, a French physician. He found that placing the woman in this position made the birth so much easier for the *doctor!*

INFANT MORTALITY AND MORBIDITY

There are far more serious consequences of orthodox obstetric methods than pain and discomfort for the mothers. The United States also makes a poor showing for safety to mother and child among nations of similar standards of living and similar culture:

> . . . Infant mortality has risen from a record low of 26 deaths per 1,000 live births in 1956 to 26.3 in 1957 to 27.1 in 1958. . . . Surprisingly, America has never ranked high in the protection offered its new born. Once in sixth place among nations, we have now fallen to tenth. Huge and rich though we are, we do not give all our mothers and babies the care they would receive in (listed in order of achievement): Sweden, Netherlands, Australia, Norway, Switzerland, Great Britain, Denmark, New Zealand, or Finland. *Not even one state within the United States can match the low infant-mortality rate reported by Sweden!* . . .
>
> For the last ten years we have made almost no progress in reducing the entire death rate (including fetal deaths) associated with childbirth. Such deaths are the fifth major cause of mortality in this country. In addition, 60,000 babies a year are damaged during birth—to survive with cerebral palsy, epilepsy, or a degree of mental crippling. (Italics added.)[11]

This is not the 1930s, or even the 1940s! In 1958, the year in which more babies died in the United States per thousand births than in nine other nations, "postnatal asphyxia and atelectasis" (imperfect expansion of the lungs at birth) was given as the leading cause of infant deaths, taking the lives of 20,395 infants. In 1960 it was still the leading cause, and provisional statistics for 1961 and 1962 showed it about tied with "all other causes" (*i.e.,* other than specified causes such as birth injury, congenital malformations, and so forth) as the leading factor in infant deaths.

By 1970 the United States had dropped to fourteenth place, although the infant mortality rate is now down to 19.8. (The infant mortality rate is based on the number of infant deaths per one thousand live births in the first year of life. Three-fourths of such deaths occur during the first few days of life.) Sweden was still in the lead, with an infant mortality rate of 11.7, and The Netherlands was still in second place, with 12.7. Added to the seven other nations with lower infant mortality rates than the United States now were Japan, Canada, France, East Germany, and Ireland.[12]

Oxygen shortage during labor or birth produces the state of

asphyxiation which can result in mental retardation, cerebral palsy, epilepsy, or death. Four major factors may leave a newborn baby short of oxygen: "Any condition which interferes with the proper exchange of oxygen and carbon dioxide between the mother and the unborn baby. Prolonged or obstructed labor. A traumatic delivery. Too high a dosage of drugs to relieve pain in labor or too deep anesthesia."[13]

Further evidence of the dangers of drugs and anesthetics in labor continues, and many physicians have warned against the misuse of these agents. Dr. Franklin F. Snyder states in the preface of his book, *Obstetric Analgesia and Anesthesia:*

> Analysis of labor from the standpoint of the child reveals the pre-eminence of fetal respiratory injury as a cause of death associated with birth. Since all drugs commonly given for the relief of pain tend to alter the functioning of respiration, thus striking the fetus at the point of maximum susceptibility to injury during labor, it is obvious that measurement of the pharmacologic factor in labor is closely linked with the detection and measurement of fetal respiratory changes. It is considerations such as these that prompt the detailed inquiry in the following pages concerning the history of the respiratory organs before birth and the principal types of pathologic alteration which involve them—asphyxia, atelectasis, and pneumonia.[14]

So the "pharmacologic factor" makes an infant more susceptible to respiratory infections. Perhaps this helps to explain the increasing death rate from such infections in the last decade. A Children's Bureau report states:

> While in general during 1950–57 decreases occurred in infant mortality from postnatal causes—such as certain infectious and parasitic diseases, diseases of the digestive system, and accidents—death rates from infections of unidentified types showed small but continuing increases. These included: *pneumonia of the newborn . . . acute upper respiratory infection, bronchitis, and related infections . . .* meningitis, except meningococcal and tuberculous . . . "other infections of the newborn," 53 per cent [increase in rate per 100,000 live births]; and septicemia and pyemia [blood poisonings],

48 per cent. . . . . Had the death rate for these causes decreased at about the pace of the death rate for infectious and parasitic diseases as a whole, the lives of approximately 2,500 infants annually in 1954–7 would have been spared. (Italics added.)[15]

The Children's Bureau is encouraging studies to determine how this increase in infections in the newborn may also be related to increased hospitalization for childbirth, since infections in central nurseries spread rapidly. This is one of the most important reasons for encouraging rooming-in.

There are other factors that contribute to lower infant mortality rates. Sweden's excellent record, for example, exists in spite of the fact that it has only 60 per cent as many doctors as the United States, based on population size. But 85 per cent of the births in Sweden and Norway are conducted by nurse-midwives. Furthermore, a large number of these births take place in the home, whereas in the United States 83 per cent of nonwhite births and 96 per cent of white births now take place in the hospital.

Socialized medicine, prenatal care, and maternity care are available in Sweden free of charge to every mother. All children are under medical supervision in child-care centers, where they receive all necessary inoculations and whatever treatment is necessary. Part of their program of socialized medicine consists of education. In all cities expectant mothers can enroll voluntarily in classes with training in natural childbirth. Courses in baby care are also available. High school girls are taught not only housekeeping and child-care methods but are also instructed in natural childbirth methods.

The disadvantage to the socialized medical program in Sweden is that while every physician and nurse-midwife is knowledgeable about natural childbirth, there is never one person who follows a woman through the pregnancy and birth. When a woman enters the hospital for the birth, she does not know which of the trained staff physicians or nurse-midwives will be her attendants.

The young wife of an exchange student, who had been trained in nursing and pediatrics in Sweden, told me that part of her training had included how to teach childbirth methods to expectant parents.

She was employed in the nursery for newborn in a large hospital while here in the United States, and when I mentioned to her that I had had three natural birth experiences, she exclaimed, "Oh, I'm so glad to hear you say that! I was beginning to think no one in the United States knew anything about natural childbirth, since no one seems to understand it here in the hospital. The new babies are brought into the nursery so drugged. I just can't understand it. I always thought the United States was ahead in everything, but I've been disillusioned."

A Scottish obstetrician remarked that members of the medical profession in his country consider the United States "hopelessly behind in its obstetric system."

But in contrast to the poor over-all American average, in an early natural childbirth program at Yale there were only thirty infant deaths of 2,024 infants delivered. And in the twenty years from 1931 to 1951, in which the New York Maternity Center was conducting home deliveries, they had

> . . . a neonatal death rate of 14 per 1,000 births or 15 per 1,000 live births. In this group there was a high incidence of poor nutrition, poor home conditions, low income, unmarried mothers, and high parity. In spite of this our neonatal death rate is much lower than the rate for the whole Clinic area.[16]

This fine record is all the more remarkable when it is realized that half of these births occurred before, or in the early days of, the development of antibiotics. And although the European methods of natural childbirth were not known during the early part of this period, the Maternity Center methods were similar to them. Ether was made available at home deliveries, but the mothers seldom wanted it. In fact, during the last nine years of the twenty-year period, it wasn't used at all, even though it was available if the mother asked for it.

In the United States as a whole, not only do too many babies die, but too many are permanently injured during birth. It has been variously estimated by specialists that 35 per cent to 70 per cent of the 60,000 birth injuries a year were preventable. Take the lowest estimate—about 35 per cent, or a little over 20,000 babies a year—and think a moment. *Twenty thousand babies unnecessarily crippled mentally or physically at birth every single year in the United States* represent more injured children than polio ever crippled in the United States in a year. According to statistics in an article by Dr. Albert B. Sabin,[17] the highest incidence of polio in the United States before 1950 occurred in 1916, when 27,363 children were stricken. But Dr. Sabin points out that often from 40 per cent to 60 per cent of reported polio cases are not paralytic.

The appalling figure of 20,000 infants unnecessarily injured at birth during a single year even *exceeds the world count of babies maimed* as a result of their mothers' having taken the drug Thalidomide during their pregnancies.

How can we accept this so complacently? Although the National Institute of Neurological Diseases and Blindness is spending more than $1 million during a ten-year period to track down the causes of cerebral palsy and mental retardation in over 40,000 children, checking the effects of heredity, oxygen shortage at birth, and injury during delivery, the use of drugs during pregnancy and labor, and maternal infections, the public at large seems apathetic.

In 1940, the *Journal of Pediatrics* reported that of a group of more than nine hundred children whose brain defects could not be traced to heredity or injury during childhood, "70 per cent were found to have a history of asphyxia, regardless of the manner of delivery or whether the baby was full term, premature, or a twin."[18]

This may have been understandable in 1940, but the same is still too true today. A neurosurgeon states that brain damage caused by lack of oxygen at birth produces more nerve disorders of the brain than hereditary factors.[19] Still another report says:

> It is now known that much feeblemindedness is directly due to a lack of oxygen during the actual birth process; anoxia can destroy brain cells in a perfectly normal child during the final moments of birth. Dr. F. W. Windle . . . has asphyxiated guinea pigs at birth in a way that simulates anoxic conditions under which infants are born. Many of the guinea pigs show obvious brain damage and aberrations of the nervous system in the period just

after birth. But often by the end of a few weeks they have lost these obvious defects and behave, to outward observation, like normal pigs. But as adults they *learn more slowly and forget more quickly* than normal animals. *"The highest brain centers were the ones most permanently damaged,"* says Dr. Windle. . . . Prolonged labor and abnormally prolonged contractions of the uterus at the time of birth are two ways in which human babies are made anoxic. One factor which can prolong labor and uterine contractions is improper use of pain-killing drugs and anesthetics during childbirth. (Italics added.)[20]

Dr. Arnold Gesell, in *Developmental Diagnosis,* explains that the danger of permanent mental disabling from anoxia is greatest for the child who may already have only a poorly developed nervous system:

A newborn ament is likely to show cyanosis of severe grade on small provocation. . . . On the other hand, an infant of superior endowment may escape some of the permanent effects which an inferior child would suffer. The well-endowed nervous system would give him greater protection.[21]

While she was on tour for the National Foundation in January 1963, Dr. Virginia Apgar, well-known authority on birth defects, revealed to her audience the startling fact that one out of every sixteen Americans has a recognizable defect (mental or physical) at birth.

Of course the misuse of analgesics and anesthetics during birth is not the only cause of mental crippling. Several other contributing factors have been identified, and there are still other causes that are not yet known.

Babies are born with physical handicaps, too, such as cerebral palsy, which is apparent a few weeks after birth. Although there are many factors contributing to the high incidence of cerebral palsy in the United States—"an estimated prevalence rate of . . . about 150 per 100,000,"[22] the American Public Health Association reports:

Factors incident to labor and birth (including sequelae in the neonatal period) are generally considered to be first in importance as a cause of cerebral palsy, prenatal factors second, and postnatal factors third.[23]

In this same booklet the following precautions are included with others: "Care in recourse to Cesarean delivery. Care in the use of obstetric analgesia and anesthesia. Careful consideration of the need for medical induction of labor."[24] And in precautions against the possibility of cerebral palsy for premature babies they warn: "Particular caution in the use of obstetric analgesia and anesthesia in premature births."[25]

Dr. C. Lee Buxton of Yale University School of Medicine also mentions the possibility of birth drugs being involved in the incidence of cerebral palsy:

The preliminary findings of the multi-disciplinary collaborative anterospective study of cerebral palsy presently being carried out in fourteen institutions in the United States indicate a possibility that anoxia may be a significant factor in brain damage, making itself evident some time after the perinatal period.[26]

The use of forceps, as well as of drugs, is also implicated as a possible cause of cerebral palsy. Dr. Winthrop M. Phelps reported in the *Cerebral Palsy Institute Proceedings* that

. . . to keep our chronological order, we then must admit that there are birth injuries due to forceps which cause pressure and a fractured skull and subdural hemorrhage. We know also that in this situation you would have cortical damage, and in all probability, spasticity.[27]

In extremely difficult and complicated births, the use of forceps may be unavoidable, even though it results in such injuries. But what about the use of forceps in normal deliveries? Another cause of cerebral palsy resulting from birth is said to be the danger of "excessive traction in a head presentation with a stretching of the neck."[28] Another doctor describes how forceps are used:

The forceps consist of two wide flat blades curved to fit gently over the child's head. The blades are inserted and brought into position separately, and are then locked together, firmly gripping the head. By turning and gently pulling the child is extracted.[29]

Is it not possible that this "turning and gently pulling" can at times create "excessive traction in a head presentation with a stretching of the neck, "which may result in cerebral palsy?" Yet we find that some physicians say that they use forceps 90 per cent of the time. They say that it is "better" for the baby than for his head to keep "pounding on the perineum." But if forceps are one of the contributing factors in the incidence of cerebral palsy, it would seem sensible to use them with much greater caution.

The late Dr. J. Lawrence Cochran called forceps "the steel hatband" in his article "Concerning Birth Injuries," which appeared in *Medical Times* in 1956. He wrote:

> How much intracranial trauma can be inflicted to the delicate structures inside the infant's calvaria by a forceps *properly* applied —not to even mention an improper application of this inflexible instrument. . . . 70% of cerebral palsy may be justly and reasonably attributed wholly to brain traumata incurred during the process of childbirth.[30]

Of course, no thinking person could ever deny that forceps are useful, essential, obstetrical tools that have saved the lives of many babies. In these instances, when a baby's life has been at stake, the risk of using them has been justifiable. But to use forceps routinely and indiscriminately in normal labors seems indefensible.

MATERNAL MORTALITY AND MORBIDITY

In the United States Vital Statistics records of maternal mortality, anesthetic deaths are not listed. These deaths are effectively hidden under listings such as "delivery without mention of complication"; "delivery complicated by prolonged labor of other origin" (*i.e.*, other than disproportion or malposition of the fetus); "delivery with other trauma"; "delivery with other complications of childbirth," and so forth. How many of these mysterious "other" causes might be attributable to anesthetics if the truth were known? In 1958 and 1959 these "other" causes were responsible for almost as many maternal deaths as were caused by hemorrhaging. And this does not even take into consideration the possibility of unnecessary hemorrhage due to the use of anesthesia. Obviously, statistics concerning anesthetic deaths should be recorded in order to pinpoint these "other" causes of maternal deaths.

In *Childbirth—with Understanding,* Dr. Herbert Thoms reports that

> . . . in 1952 in New York City, anesthesia was the cause of maternal mortality in fifth place behind hemorrhage, infection, toxemia and heart disease. . . . Fitzgerald and Webster reporting in 1953, found that 44 per cent of all maternal deaths in three St. Louis hospitals were from anesthesia.[31]

But even in areas where anesthetic deaths are listed as such, they are often unreported or are falsely listed under some other heading. This is made very plain in a report on the results of studies in maternal mortality in Minnesota, which have been conducted every year since 1950:

> A number of surprising things were uncovered. There was often a positive diagnosis on the death certificate when none was possible. . . . In circumstances where no diagnosis was possible, a physician supplied one from a fertile imagination because "If I don't, the death certificate will be returned to me and I don't want to be bothered." An occasional diagnosis was falsified. . . . Pulmonary embolism is blamed for all manner of things with which it has nothing whatever to do. . . .
>
> This has quite effectively hidden a great many significant factors in maternal deaths. *Perhaps the best example of this is the significance of the injudicious use of spinal anesthesia which is seldom given as a cause of death.* The problem of the risk of obstetric anesthesia becomes very clear from a detailed study such as this. Over the same time period in Minnesota there were 10 deaths from obstetric anesthesia and 13 deaths from eclampsia. There seems to be a lesson here. . . .

If one combines the totals of death certificates of maternal deaths which did not list a recent obstetric event and those which carried an incorrect diagnosis of cause of death in 1951 . . . the combined error of missed cases and incorrect diagnosis was . . . 41.3 per cent. Under any circumstances the error is large. . . .

In the absence of a detailed study, maternal mortality data as they are usually collected and reported are not reliable since the material on which they are based is grossly inaccurate. (Italics added.)[32]

General anesthesia, as well as spinal anesthesia, carries the risk of death to the mother. An article titled "Obstetrical Analgesia and Anesthesia," which appeared in the *Journal of the American Medical Association* in 1957, explains why:

Unlike the patient prepared for surgery, most women in labor have food in their stomachs. . . . Aspiration of vomitus is one of the greatest hazards in these patients. This cause, spinal shock, and cardiac arrest account for 69% of the anesthetic deaths incurred by obstetric patients. . . . If spinal, caudal or epidural anesthesia are used it is necessary to keep close watch on the mother's blood pressure, as shock may occur suddenly. Conduction anesthesia carries the further risk of causing meningitis, epidural abscess, or arachnoiditis. . . . *No method of anesthesia is absolutely safe.* (Italics added.)[33]

The "aspiration of vomitus" mentioned here is a common cause of maternal deaths, as is demonstrated in a report as follows:

In one survey of 8330 maternal deaths quoted by the doctors, almost half were due to aspiration. . . . Forty-five additional deaths were due to over-dosage with spinal anesthesia. . . . Nearly two-thirds of these deaths were preventable.[34]

There is another unfortunate result of the use of anesthetics and drugs, and that is the depression which commonly follows childbirth. This depression is seen in the majority of American women who have had orthodox deliveries, but seldom occurs among primitive women or after an adequate natural birth experience. This depression after an orthodox delivery is understandable if real suffering has been involved and the woman feels resentful toward her child. Florence Blake describes this unhappiness as she has seen it occur:

> When the mother has experienced intense discomfort during labor and has required deep sedation and anesthesia there is more apt to be a lag in the development of emotional feelings of motherliness. The majority of these women awaken uncomfortable, fearful and unaware of what has happened to them. They have heard no birth cry and have had no opportunity to hold the child who was once an integral part of them. They have experienced no positive emotional response which has reassured them of oneness with their child. They often feel no love—only a deep sense of loss and emptiness which disturbs them and threatens their peace of mind. . . . It is difficult for these mothers to feel that their babies belong to them.[35]

Eugene Marais, the South American naturalist, experimented with anesthesia on deer and reported strikingly similar results. In a study of a herd of sixty half-wild Kaffir buck for fifteen years he saw no case in which a mother refused her young under normal conditions. But when, as an experiment, he gave anesthesia to six animals, rendering them unconscious during the birth of their offspring, *each of the six refused to accept her own lamb* and had to be coaxed to do so![36]

Dr. James Clark Moloney, a psychiatrist, says that "depression" following childbirth, if it were simply the "fatigue" which follows any exertion or tiring experience, would be cured by resting. But he reminds the reader that resting

> . . . does not cure or does not eliminate this type of exhaustion, which is a part of a depression syndrome. . . . There is always, to every mental depression, the same internal, central core. . . . This central core is a core of being resentful, of being angry, a core of being bitter. . . . I do not even like to use the term "postpartal depression," because that is affixing a name to it which rightfully does not belong there. . . . Very often the woman is not at all aware of the anger, the resentment, the bitterness behind her mental depression. . . . I wish to make this point clear because I

want to indicate as clearly as possible, with as much emphasis as possible, that there is nothing peculiar in the mental depression that should allow this condition to be connected with childbirth. I want, first and foremost, to rob the cliché of the so-called "third-day depression" of any element of physiological consistency. There is no physiological responsibility behind a mental depression. A mental depression is a psychological manifestation and it is a complete trend of events that takes place as a result of frustration.[37]

There are frustrations for a new mother caused by a painful labor, worry over an apparent inability to breast-feed, or by homesickness for her other children. But none of these even begins to explain the thousands of times this unhappiness occurs following an "easy" birth, which the mother scarcely remembers and which she was not allowed to feel; nor does it explain the thousands of times this depression occurs, sometimes with increasing severity, following the birth of a second, or third, or fourth child. The mother's frustration has no obvious reason.

There is a hormonal change in the mother that can cause a mild, temporary spell of the "blues," although this is often absent in the natural childbirth mother. The estrogen-progesterone level that has risen gradually during the pregnancy drops sharply on about the third day, about the time the milk comes in. This hormonal change can make a mother feel restless, similar to premenstrual tension. If she needs a good cry, it will help clear the air.

If the "blues" continue, however, it is well to look for more serious causes. One of these may be a change in thyroid activity,[38] which should be carefully checked by a physician if the depression lasts more than a few days.

The most important contributing factor to a continuing depression following childbirth is a subconscious feeling of being robbed, a sense of loss. For nine months of pregnancy and several hours of labor, a woman has been gradually brought to a peak of emotional and physical expectation. An adequate emotional and physical climax at the moment of birth provides a most essential catharsis for this pent-up emotion. This climax, of which one mother said,

"What an exhilarating sensation!" and another, "It was the most tremendous orgasm!" and which still another described as "a sensation of glowing warmth and comfort that is hard to describe!" is a most important part of childbearing. As the birth is completed, the sudden release, the change in physical sensations, is so dramatic, so profound, that one reacts to the sudden change and the sight of the child by laughing, or crying, or both at the same time.

This climax is essential. A mother who has missed it and had a passive, frigid birth, due to anesthetics, local injections, or hypnosis, still is emotionally in a state of expectancy. She looks at her child, but experiences no euphoria, no sense of exhilaration. But a release from pent-up emotion must come! If an adequate birth climax does not provide it, it will come later, in spells of frustrated weeping, like the tantrums of frustration of the small child who cannot explain, and indeed does not know, what it is he wants. The most adequate analogy to the depression of the new mother is the depression of the young wife who has been repeatedly aroused to a point of expectation but never fully satisfied in intercourse. She lies awake weeping in the dark, while her husband, completely satisfied, snores peacefully beside her.

A new mother does not understand why she feels such a "letdown," nor is she aware that giving birth was meant to be a most satisfying sexual experience as well as a most rewarding spiritual one. It is with difficulty that she identifies herself with her child at first, although this comes in time. She touches him gingerly, unbelievingly.

For the "natural childbirth" mother, identification with her child was not broken at birth. She looks with awe at this infant who was harbored so long within herself, recalls with keen pleasure the pleasant sensation of his warm, little body moving from her own, and he seems to her an extension of her own being. She feels no sense of loss, and this identification with her child continues as he grows. She laughs when he laughs, glows with maternal pride over each of his little achievements—holding up his head, his first tooth, his first word, his first step, and when he cries because of bumps and bruises, she weeps over him as if she herself had been hurt.

HYPNOSIS

An awareness of the serious consequences of the misuse of drugs and anesthetics for both mother and baby, combined with the erroneous medical tradition that normal childbirth is always a painful experience, has left the reflective physician with only one plausible solution: hypnosis.

Since World War II hypnosis has come into its own in the medical profession and is now an accepted method of treating both psychiatric and psychosomatic disorders, and experiments are being made regarding its value in treating certain functional disorders as well. It is also being used for anesthetic purposes— desensitizing certain areas of the body for operative purposes, so that no pain is felt. Because hypnosis carries no medicinal hazards to either mother or child, and because it makes it possible for the mother to be "awake" and still give birth to her child without pain, it is also being used for childbirth.

There are two basic misconceptions concerning hypnosis and childbirth, however. The first is that all successful natural births are due to some type of hypnosis, and the second is that hypnosis in obstetrics is to be preferred over natural childbirth, which is equated with "stoicism."

Natural childbirth, without sedation, and without pain, should not be confused with hypnotism. Dr. Edmund Jacobson has developed an apparatus (aided by the Bell Telephone Laboratories) that can test the contraction or relaxation of muscles electrically with the utmost precision—with an error of only about 0.25 millionth of a volt, so that the slightest contraction of a muscle is immediately indicated. By means of these electromyographic tests, which Dr. Jacobson calls *electroneuromyometry,* he is able to prove conclusively whether a patient who feels no pain is actually relaxed or "hypnotized." He says:

> . . . In hypnoidal states, the patient told to relax further may instead show an increase of action potentials, contrary to the efforts of the hypnotist and contrary to the claims made by the

patient that he feels more relaxed. Indeed, hypnosis cannot be relied upon to produce relaxation, being characterized often by increased action potentials and by persistence or increase of knee jerk. . . . The hypnotized patient and the patient in any form of hypnoidal trance may believe that he is relaxing and the doctor may concur; but adequate electromyographic tests disclose the contrary, as has been shown in my laboratory.[39]

Nor is a natural birth without pain due to "autosuggestion." In *Hypnotism Today* the authors say of autosuggestion: "One's frame of mind must be positive in giving suggestions, but to receive and act on these one must be completely negative. It is impossible to be both at the same time."[40]

Dr. Jacobson says of autosuggestion that it ". . . not only is not necessary; it can awaken fear by countersuggestion. A person who uses autosuggestion, whatever his purposes, is a disturbed person."[41]

There are several drawbacks to the use of hypnosis in obstetrics in place of natural childbirth.

1. *It takes too much time to employ.* LeCron and Bordeaux, in their interesting and authoritative book write that hypnotism

. . . can be produced by today's methods in about one person out of three or four and even then it may not be complete. . . . Several sessions with most subjects are needed before it can be brought out. . . . A real disadvantage is that only a small percentage of expectant mothers are good enough hypnotic subjects for the induction of complete anesthesia.[42]

2. *The "transference of affection" involved in hypnosis creates too much emotional dependence on the doctor.* The phenomenon of a woman "falling in love" with her obstetrician, to her consternation and embarrassment, is frequently mentioned in American culture. It occurs because she is ignorant of her role in childbirth, and so is emotionally dependent upon him to help her. Hypnosis increases this emotional dependence. It is essential for the hypnotist to establish such "rapport" with his patient that *all other influences are excluded.* LeCron and Bordeaux give as an example of this rapport the small girl who would not even answer her own mother while under hypnosis.

. . . This hypnotic rapport automatically establishes positive trans-ference unless neurotic factors prevent. The whole relationship between the patient and the hypnotist becomes influenced by a combination of hypnotic, neurotic, and natural tendencies, de-pending on the particular case.[43]

This "transference" is defined as a patient transferring to the therapist his affections, dependence, or hostility, sometimes with a sexual attachment.[44] This transference of affections must be re-solved if there are not to be lasting emotional repercussions after-ward. But why complicate the problem in the sexual experience of childbirth by involving the doctor in the woman's emotions at all?

Dr. Jacobson agrees that hypnotism increases "personal depend-ence, suggestibility, and neurotic symptoms,"[45] and says:

> Relaxation methods cultivate self-confidence, emotional stability, and freedom of will. . . . Hypnosis, on the contrary, favors domi-nance by the hypnotist . . . her emotions are at the hypnotists's behest. . . . A relaxed mother does not follow commands but guides her own conduct in complete freedom. She is not unduly open to any form of suggestion, but employs her energies eco-nomically and intelligently for her own purposes.[46]

3. *Hypnoanesthesia eliminates some of the benefits of an ade-quate physical and emotional climax.* Dr. Ralph W. August, in his excellent book, *Hypnosis in Obstetrics; Obstetric Hypnoanesthesia,* states as the purpose of hypnosis, the loss of sensation: "I tell my patients that my primary objective in ultilization of hypnosis is anesthesia for the delivery."[47]

Thus the hypnotized mother, like the mother given a pudendal, saddle, or similar regional nerve block, is "awake," but watches the doctor lift her child from her unfeeling body, as a magician might lift a rabbit from a hat. She doesn't suffer, but neither does she "enjoy" the sensations of the birth. Dr. Buxton mentions that

> . . . as a method for pain relief in labor and delivery it [hypnosis] may be considered to have the advantage of an elimination of the possible dangers of pharmacological analgesia and anesthesia, but

it does not, however, permit a woman to participate in the process of labor and delivery nor provide her with the satisfaction, sense of accomplishment, and "joy of birth" which are provided by other methods and which are said to be such valuable contributions to psychological health and equanimity.[48]

Dr. August points out certain disadvantages in hypnoanesthesia:

> Its use may present problems. Its misuse may lead to serious difficulties for both patient and physician. . . . It is true that care must be taken in order that an overt psychosis not be precipitated in a patient disposed toward psychosis. . . . Some anxious or prepsychotic patients may accept hypnotically created fantasy as reality. There are some who may fear removal of symbolic defenses.[49]

Dr. August's willingness to admit that hypnosis may present certain problems, and his congenial, nondogmatic manner concerning its use in obstetrics, are a welcome and refreshing change. His patients are free to refuse hypnosis if they wish. However, if employed by physicians like Dr. August, who are thoroughly trained in its proper application and do not insist upon it as the "only way," hypnosis for childbirth will retain a solid place in future obstetrics. One of its distinct advantages is that it fills the gap between the dangers of anesthesia and the inability of some mothers to have natural childbirth, owing to physical abnormalities or reluctance to try. Dr. August says:

> Hypnosis is of particular value to the poor-risk mother, the patient with cardiac, renal or pulmonary disease, the debilitated patient, the one with multiple allergies. . . . It is the only absolutely safe anesthetic for both mother and baby. It is the only one which has never yet been listed as a cause of death.[50]

CONCLUSION

The joy inherent in a natural birth is a philosophy that represents a universal truth. But the *application* of that philosophy must of necessity be on an individual basis. Hazel Corbin, director of the Maternity Center Association, reminds us that

> each person is an individual with her own anatomical and physiological and psychological makeup, in a socio-economic group with cultural patterns and customs. All of these factors can influence the outcome of pregnancy and labor. . . . Each mother's performance is conditioned by her background and the care she gets through pregnancy and labor.

In Europe, childbirth is conducted in a more humane manner than is customary in the United States, and a satisfying birth experience is looked upon as a woman's right. This is true even in areas where education for natural childbirth is still not available. A physician from Holland compares a European delivery with one in an American hospital:

> I must say that when I came here, when I came into the OB department, the very first days I was shocked. What I saw was women brought into the delivery room in quite a few instances, hurry, hurry, hurry—everybody seemed quite excited because as soon as possible they prepared the delivery room. Then the mother was washed very quickly and masks put on. The obstetrician prepared himself. Then the forceps were put on, rather often—much more often than we do it over in Holland—and the baby was delivered with one of the nurses pushing on the abdomen—and dragged by the obstetrician out of the mother. I was shocked because in Holland home deliveries have a kind of, I would say, cozy atmosphere and everything is much more quiet. People know each other and the doctor and, in a lot of cases, the maternity nurse, and the woman is just lying in her bed where she is every day—every night, I should say—. She feels much more relaxed and the father is around. One of the bigger daughters, maybe, is around and everything is much more human. . . . I didn't find this at all in delivery rooms with shining objects all around. This makes a big difference.[51]

Mothers would like to see more of this "humanization" in maternity care. Many of us, like myself, have had happy natural birth experiences without receiving any encouragement—not to say in the face of open skepticism—from the doctors who attended us. But we have not lost faith in the medical profession. We are most grateful for those outstanding physicians who have the courage to provide leadership in the desperately needed reforms in our obstetrical systems. We are confident that increasing numbers of physicians will also assume such leadership as they become aware of the benefits of natural childbirth to mother and baby, and will help educate women everywhere for such wholesome birth experiences. We fully believe that obstetricians will become determined to keep their pledge to the Hippocratic oath more fully in their practice of obstetrics in the years just ahead:

> I will prescribe regimen for the good of my patients according to my ability and my judgment and never do harm to anyone. To please no one will I prescribe a deadly drug, nor give advice which may cause his death. . . . If I keep this oath faithfully, may I enjoy my life and practice my art, respected by all men and in all times; but if I swerve from it or violate it, may the reverse be my lot.

Notes

1. Howard W. Haggard, M.D., *Devils, Drugs, and Doctors: The Story of the Science of Healing from Medicine Man to Doctor* (New York: Harper, 1929), pp. 119, 120.
2. C. Lee Buxton, M.D., *A Study of Psychophysical Methods for Relief of Childbirth Pain* (Philadelphia: Saunders, 1962), pp. 1, 2, 3. Reprinted by permission.
3. *Ibid.,* p. 14.
4. Herbert Ratner, M.D., "Medicine." One of a series of interviews on the American character by the Center for the Study of Democratic Institutions, pp. 27, 28. Reprinted by permission.
5. Quoted in "Too Many Babies Die," Margaret Hickey, *Ladies Home Journal*, August 1961, p. 140. Reprinted by special permission of *The Ladies' Home Journal*, Coypright 1961. Curtis Publishing Company.
6. Herbert Thoms, M.D., *Childbirth—With Understanding* (Springfield, Ill.: Charles C. Thomas, 1962), p. 16. Reprinted by permission.
7. Herbert Thoms, M.D., and Emil D. Karlovsky, M.D., "Two Thou-

sand Deliveries Under Training for Childbirth Program," *American Journal of Obstetrics and Gynecology* (St. Louis: C. V. Mosby Co.), Vol. 68.1, July 1954, pp. 281 283. Reprinted by permission.

8. A statement of William K. Rashbaum, M.D., in the panel discussion "Group Approaches to Childbirth Education," printed in the *ICEA 1962 Conference Report*, p. 83. Reprinted by permission.

9. Isadore B. Fogel, M.D., "The Enema—Is It Necessary?" *American Journal of Obstetrics and Gynecology* (St. Louis: C. V. Mosby Co.), Vol. 84.1, September 15, 1962, pp. 825, 830. Reprinted by permission.

10. Niles Newton, *Maternal Emotions* (New York: Hoeber, Harper, 1955). Reprinted by permission.

11. Hickey, "Too Many Babies Die," p. 43. Reprinted by permission.

12. Doris Haire, "The Cultural Warping of Childbirth," ICEA *News*, Vol. 11, No. 1.

13. Robert N. Kelso, M.D., "First Minutes of Life Termed Most Critical," *Child-Family Digest*, September-October 1960, p. 73. Reprinted by permission.

14. Franklin F. Snyder, M.D., *Obstetric Analgesia and Anesthesia* (Philadelphia: Saunders, 1949), pp. v, vi. Reprinted by permission.

15. Alice D. Chenoweth, M.D., and Eleanor P. Hunt, Ph.D., *Current Trends in Infant Mortality*, reproduced by the United States Department of Health, Education and Welfare, Social Security Administration, Children's Bureau, from *Children*, November-December 1960, p. 215.

16. Marion D. Laird, M.D., "Report of Maternity Center Clinic," *American Journal of Obstetrics and Gynecology* (St. Louis, C. V. Mosby Co.), Vol. 69.1, p. 184. Reprinted by permission.

17. Albert B. Sabin, M.D., "Epidemiologic Patterns of Poliomyelitis in Different Parts of the World," *Poliomyelitis* (Philadelphia: Lippincott, 1949), pp. 3–31.

18. Frederick Schreiber, M.D., "Neurologic Sequelae of Paranatal Asphyxia," *Journal of Pediatrics* (St. Louis, C. V. Mosby Co.), Vol. 16, 1940, p. 301. Reprinted by permission.

19. J. Lawrence Cochran, M.D., "Concerning Birth Injuries," *Medical Times*, Vol. 84, 1956, pp. 1336–1340.

20. Gladys Denny Schultz, "The Uninsulted Child," *Ladies' Home Journal*, June 1956. Reprinted by permission.

21. Arnold Gesell, M.D., and C. S. Amatruda, M.D., *Developmental Diagnosis*, 2nd ed. (New York: Hoeber, Harper, 1948), pp. 217–219.

22. *Services for Children with Cerebral Palsy*, sponsored by the Com-

mittee on Child Health of the American Public Health Association and the American Academy for Cerebral Palsy (Copyright, 1955, by the American Public Health Association, Inc.), p. 13. Reprinted by permission.
23. *Ibid.*, p. 19. Reprinted by permission.
24. *Ibid.*, p. 20. Reprinted by permission.
25. *Ibid.*, p. 20. Reprinted by permission.
26. Buxton, *A Study of Psychophysical Methods for Relief of Childbirth Pain*, p. 9. Reprinted by permission.
27. Winthrop Morgan Phelps, M.D., "Etiology and Diagnostic Classification of Cerebral Palsy," *Cerebral Palsy Institute Proceedings* (New York: Coordinating Council for Cerebral Palsy in New York City, 1950), p. 5. Reprinted by permission.
28. *Ibid.*, p. 5.
29. Haggard, *Devils, Drugs, and Doctors*, p. 54.
30. Cochran, "Concerning Birth Injuries," pp. 1336, 1338. Reprinted by permission.
31. Thoms, *Childbirth with Understanding*, pp. 11, 12. Reprinted by permission
32. J. L. McKelvey, M.D., and D. W. Freeman, M.D., "Critical Evaluation of the Minnesota Maternal Mortality Study," *American Journal of Obstetrics and Gynecology* (St. Louis: C. V. Mosby Co.), Vol. 68.1, July 1954, pp. 30, 31, 32, 37. Reprinted by permission.
33. Snyder, "Obstetric Analgesia and Anesthesia," *Journal of the American Medical Association*, Vol. 165, No. 17, p. 2198. Reprinted by permission.
34. Reported in *Child-Family Digest*, September 1952. Reprinted by permission.
35. Florence G. Blake, R.N., M.A., *The Child, His Parents and the Nurse* (Philadelphia: Lippincott, 1954), p. 73. Reprinted by permission.
36. Eugene Marais, *The Soul of the White Ant* (New York: Dodd, Mead, 1937).
37. James Clark Moloney, M.D., "Post-Partum Depression or Third-Day Depression Following Childbirth," *Child-Family Digest*, February 1952, pp. 21–23. Reprinted by permission.
38. Virginia Larsen, M.D., *Prediction and Improvement of Postpartum Adjustment* (Fort Steilacoom, Wash.: Division of Research, 1968).
39. Edmund Jacobson, M.D., *How to Relax and Have Your Baby* (New York: McGraw-Hill, 1959), pp. 176, 180. Reprinted by permission.

40. Leslie M. LeCron, Ph.D., and Jean Bordeaux, Ph.D., *Hypnotism Today* (New York: Grune and Stratton, 1947), p. 135.
41. Jacobson, *How to Relax and Have Your Baby,* p. 145. Reprinted by permission.
42. LeCron, *Hypnotism Today,* pp. 109, 249, 250.
43. *Ibid.,* p. 218.
44. *Ibid.,* pp. 190 ff.
45. Jacobson, *How to Relax and Have Your Baby,* p. 187. Reprinted by permission.
46. *Ibid.,* pp. 14–16. Reprinted by permission.
47. Ralph V. August, M.D., *Hypnosis in Obstetrics: Obstetric Hypno-anesthesia* (New York: McGraw-Hill, Blakiston Division, 1961), p. 144. Reprinted by permission.
48. Buxton, *A Study of Psychophysical Methods for Relief of Childbirth Pain, p.* 54. Reprinted by permission.
49. August, *Hypnosis in Obstetrics,* pp. 144, 145. Reprinted by permission.
50. *Ibid.,* p. 146. Reprinted by permission.
51. A statement made in the panel discussion "Approaches to Childbirth Around the World," *ICEA 1962 Convention Report,* p. 5. Reprinted by permission.

Chapter 20

Family-Centered Maternity Care

EDUCATION FOR CHILDBIRTH

The importance of adequate education for childbirth cannot be overestimated. Expectant young couples, in today's intelligent societies, are eager for such education and respond to it with enthusiasm. But facts concerning the physical processes of sex reproduction are not enough. Far more important is the instilling of the right attitudes toward both mating and childbirth as God-given privileges and blessings.

Ideally, the instilling of right attitudes should begin in the home when the child is small. He is affected, through actions if not through words, by the attitudes prevalent in the family in which he is growing up. Too often the home fails to provide him with either the factual information or the positive attitudes he needs. Thus sex education is left to the schools and childbirth education is left to the hospitals.

Churches are finally beginning to become aware of their responsibilities to families in this important aspect of their lives. Many churches are now providing sex education for their young people, *along with* the instilling of Christian attitudes toward it. Courses for young married couples in marriage and the family are also beginning to appear in the churches. Education for childbirth can hardly be omitted in such courses. And it is here that the presentation of childbirth as God's wonderful plan for the completion of the Christian home belongs. God's plan assures a welding of the bond between husband and wife as co-creators of a "family."

For information on good materials for childbirth education, both for individuals and for groups, the reader is referred to Appendix A.

THE HUSBAND'S ROLE

There is one caricature in contemporary publications that is familiar to all of us. This is the caricature of the helpless, jittery male pacing the waiting-room floor, or reading a magazine upside down, as he waits for his wife to give birth to their child beyond the doors which read NO ADMITTANCE.

Medical personnel and hospital administrators are aghast at the thought of bringing this helpless, jittery creature into the sacrosanct "halls of birth."

But why is the poor fellow helpless and jittery? With a little training, so he understands what is taking place and what he can do to help, he can be an indispensable asset to his wife in both the labor and delivery rooms. One husband explains the expectant father's role in this way:

> Unluckily, a lot of things make it pretty hard for a woman to just take it easy and let labor run its course. There are old wives' tales, the talk about descending into the valley of death, the atmosphere of terror, which surround childbirth. There is the hospital atmosphere, the hospital odor, the glimpses of sheeted figures being wheeled along the corridors. There are the grimly cheerless labor rooms, and the faces of strangers peering over the guardrail—kindly faces, maybe, but nevertheless strange ones. There is the lurking thought that something, after all, may go seriously wrong. . . .
>
> So far as I can see, and I've seen it, the only relaxing elements in this routine are the shot in the arm and the few capsules they give a patient to swallow.
>
> That's where the expectant father comes in—or should come in. His wife, no matter how "medicated," will see and recognize him as a familiar, reassuring face in an otherwise alarmingly alien

place. She'll see him as a guy who's going to be right there all the time, and not just as a genie of the press-button device.

A man doesn't need to be a miracle worker to play his role to perfection. *He merely needs to be there. Period.*[1]

One of the chief criticisms of modern obstetrics is the "loneliness" of the long hours of the first stage of labor. For this reason, the importance of "support during labor" is currently being emphasized. But who is most capable of giving this "support"? One doctor says:

> . . . We have never yet found a companion that beats a husband for the simple reason that they love each other. What is he going to do? He is going to reassure his wife and guide her and coach her in relaxation, we have found by actual practice. I think it would be much simpler for us to hire some woman—pick one of our physiotherapists and hire her to sit with our patient—we tried that, and it doesn't work worth a hoot, for the simple reason that I haven't found a woman yet who will, under stress particularly, pay much attention to the advice of another woman. "Who's that old bat think she is to be telling me what to do?" we found sometimes was a subconscious, if not a conscious attitude, of our patients towards the attendant; but we found that husbands are magnificent teachers of relaxation. . . . The familiarity of an ever loving husband's voice is the most soothing relaxing thing on earth to a patient, particularly when this patient knows that *this father to be knows what he is doing. He has been trained.* (Italics added.)[2]

Many hospitals are letting down their barriers and permitting husbands in the labor rooms. But the same old rule still applies to too many delivery rooms. The wife is wheeled in, and the door is shut in the husband's face. What kind of Victorian prudery is this? Is the arrival of a new son or daughter into the world such a vulgar sight that the father of the child should not see it? Is the wife to be subjected to such horrors in the hands of the medical attendants that it is better for the husband not to know about it? These are some of the questions in his mind as he waits outside the closed door.

Some hospitals provide "amphitheaters" where the husband may observe the birth from beyond a glass. What a revolting thought! A husband does not want to be present as a "spectator," as if the birth were a "spectacle." His curiosity as to how a birth takes place should already have been satisfied through films, books, and pictures. His place during the birth is not beyond a cold glass, but by his wife's side, supporting her when she pushes, whispering words of encouragement in her ear, and letting her see the love in his eyes.

The argument that the husband will "contaminate" the sterile room, is invalid. Soap and water are cheap, aren't they? And there are plenty of sterile caps and gowns around.

Sometimes the nurses are embarrassed by the presence of the husbands, and don't quite know what to do with them. In *Family-Centered Maternity Nursing*,[3] Ernestine Wiedenbach explains how the nurse can be at ease with the men around, and how to help make this a happy "shared" experience for the husband and wife.

Some doctors have worried about the effect on husbands if something "goes wrong" at the birth. Husbands who *have* been present in such an emergency, and who have lost a child, say that they were most grateful to have been there. This way they realized that every possible attempt was made to save their baby. Otherwise, they say they might always have thought that the baby was lost through some negligence of the attendants.

Dr. Bradley of Denver, Colorado, has delivered over several thousand babies with the husband present throughout labor and delivery. In a recent issue of *Psychosomatics,* in an article entitled "Fathers' Presence in Delivery Rooms," he explains why he feels that a trained husband is an important member of the "birth team;" and answers some of the common objections to the husbands being present. He says, for example, that husbands do not "get in the way." They are placed next to their wives and disturb no one. He says that husbands do not get sick or faint, having been prepared by special classes during their wives' pregnancies; and they wear sterile gowns so there is no danger on that score. Dr. Bradley also has sensible answers to the two most serious objections:

What if there are unforeseen "complications"? . . . Complications are exceedingly rare to begin with (96.4 per cent of vaginal deliveries are spontaneous births). However, when they occur, completely honest exp'anations are made to the parents at the time, and their assistance elicited. . . . A forceps bruise on a baby will be far better accepted by a husband who, by his presence, clearly saw the lack of progress necessitating the forceps, than a bewildered, doubtful husband who, by his absence, imagines all sorts of mismanagement. . . .

What if the baby were deformed? For this exceedingly rare occurrence we have no way of "keeping it from" the parents. . . . In the absence of anesthetic depression of the mother we feel there is no contra-indication to complete honesty to both parents at birth.

In our opinion it would be a crime to deprive thousands of the joy of seeing their normal babies at birth in order to postpone the inevitable stress of the exceedingly few with abnormal infants.[4]

A husband who was with his wife during the birth of their child describes his experience in this way:

I have just been the witness to a miracle—the awe-inspiring miracle of birth. . . . It was unforgettable. For it was the birth of my own child. I was sharing with my wife the beginning of life.

I had been spared the endless pacing of a hospital corridor, the haunted stares at closed ward doors, the agonizing doubts. Instead, I held my wife's hand as our baby was born. . . .

The first stage of birth lasted 12 hours and was no ordeal. In fact, Vera enjoyed it. It ended at 10 o'clock on a recent Sunday morning. Then I was dressed in white and taken to my wife.

She welcomed me with a smile and said she felt wonderful. I stood at her side and took her hand. We joked with the nurse, the doctor and students as that hour fled painlessly by—joked because even laughter is not out of place in this hospital's delivery rooms. . . . And eventually we saw the entry into this world of our son.

A birth had been concluded—a birth without anesthetic, pain or frightfulness. My wife tells me that for her it was unbelievably wonderful. I shall never forget her smile. I shall never forget the birth of our son. I know it brought us closer together than we have ever been before.[5]

Of course, it must be realized that there are times when a husband might not want to be with his wife, or when she would not want him there. It is no more rational to insist that *every* husband must be in the delivery room with his wife than it is to insist that every husband must be kept out. The majority of young people who have had natural childbirth training want very much to be together and should be permitted this privilege. A few, for reasons of their own, do not want it. But as one wife said, "At least it's nice to have a choice!"

One young wife said recently of her natural childbirth experience: "My happiness would have been complete if my husband had been permitted to share this beautiful moment." Another natural childbirth mother told of her husband's disappointment at being barred from the delivery room: He felt "he'd been deprived of one of the greatest spiritual experiences that can come to a father—that of seeing his own child born. . . . My joy, then, was dimmed a little, as I felt his disappointment—the unfairness of it all. After all, had we not shared equally in the creation of this child? Was not this little daughter literally his very own flesh and blood and life and breath? How could he, the father, have contaminated the delivery room any more than I, the mother? We were co-creators, neither of us more 'sterile' than the other!"[6]

HOME BIRTHS

Ninety-six per cent of all white births, and 83 per cent of all nonwhite births in the United States take place in hospitals, because home births are not considered safe. Yet when mothers have been carefully selected for home births, referring to the hospital any in whom a possible complication is suspected, statistics show that home births, under adequate medical supervision, can be safe.

The usual procedure is to have the mother supply all the essentials for herself and the baby, while the attending physician brings his own clinic bag and medicine kit. Apparatus for treating complications is either right at hand or readily available, including a portable oxygen tank and incubator, and apparatus for blood transfusion.

The biggest single worry in a home birth is postpartum hemorrhage, which may occur suddenly and profusely. Yet the Maternity Center Association of New York City, delivering 4,988 women at home over a twenty-year period, lost not one single mother due to postpartum hemorrhage, although this occurred in 4.3 per cent of the births. As soon as the bleeding was controlled the mother was given infusions of dextrose. If transfusions were necessary, she was transferred to the hospital.

The Chicago Maternity Center, which also delivered thousands of babies in the poorest of homes, lost *not a single mother* from any cause during a sequence of 12,106 deliveries. During that same period of time the national average was one maternal death for every five hundred babies born. During a three-year period in the 1950's, nine thousand consecutive home births were conducted by the Center without a single maternal death.

Part of the success of these home birth programs was due to the use of well-qualified nurse-midwives. Delores Henne, a certified nurse-midwife, describes her experiences in delivering babies at home:

> From February to June [1956], I did home deliveries in the cosmopolitan city of New York, chiefly among Puerto Rican mothers of whom many spoke only Spanish. Home deliveries are unique. The children have the advantage of seeing the baby shortly after delivery, and what a thrill it is to see their interest and enthusiasm in their new baby brother or sister. The father is given the opportunity to stay and to encourage his wife during labor and delivery. And mother has the advantage of rooming-in, having the baby with her in the same room.[7]

In thirteen other countries of the world where nurse-midwives are widely employed in delivering babies, very frequently at home, statistics show that fewer babies die per thousand live births than in the United States, where babies are delivered almost exclusively by doctors in hospitals! In these other countries home births are still looked on with favor. Gillian Mitchell, a midwife from England explains why:

> Childbirth is a normal and natural event and every effort is made to encourage this concept in England. Classes are held for mothers where they can get advice from health visitors concerning diet and exercises. . . .
>
> In England, as in Holland, the birth of the baby can take place either in the hospital or in the home. It is conceded that the home is the ideal place for the woman to have the baby. They feel that relaxation is easier here and the risk of infection is reduced to a minimum. And the bond between the mother and the baby is more securely nurtured.[8]

Dr. Oliver Hayward, a general practitioner in New Hampshire for twenty-five years, wrote in a personal letter to Dr. Thoms:

> After coming to New Hampshire I had a moderately busy obstetrical practice delivering from 12 to 20 cases a year and until the war at least half of them were delivered at home. I found that far and away the most important element in home deliveries was psychological. The patient was not sick and therefore not interested in going to the hospital, but was well and staying at home to have a baby. The presence of her husband, anxious to help and comforting in his understanding certainly relieved a great deal of tension which makes for pain. The presence of her children around the home was reassuring. . . . Another important point in home delivery was that the mechanics of the situation make it more difficult to interfere obstetrically. It is unwise and hasty obstetrical interference which causes an appreciable amount of the difficulty that I see. . . .
>
> The problem is to translate the good things of home delivery to the hospital, i.e., with rooming-in and the presence of the husband in the labor and delivery rooms.[9]

In his new book, *The Humanization of Man*,[10] Ashley Montagu suggests one solution to the problem of dealing with emergencies that might occur in a home birth. He suggests that each community should have fully equipped mobile birth units that could be stationed outside a home during the birth of a baby, ready to aid in any emergency, or, in extreme cases, to transfer the patient to the hospital. In England, fully equipped "Flying Squads" such as he describes, have been available for years.

During the early 1970's there has been an increasing trend in the United States toward giving birth at home. Young couples in both "hippie" communes and in the more traditional, middle-class areas of society are rebelling against being robbed of the right to have their children born in the dignity and peace of their own homes.

Responsible physicians are urging the medical profession to take serious note of this trend by making hospital care more homelike and by giving young couples the right to determine the manner in which the birth is to be conducted, rather than forcing them into the "routine" obstetric pattern.

It is not likely that a great many American mothers will have the privilege of a home birth under present circumstances. The doctors don't have the time, they don't have the necessary equipment, and many communities don't have the necessary emergency equipment readily available if problems should arise. But this is something we can work for. Dr. Montagu points out that mobile birth units would be far less expensive to maintain and service than fire trucks and would also be much less costly than a hospital stay. With the development of such mobile units and with an increase in the number of fully qualified nurse-midwives, home births could once again become the happy privilege of many American mothers.

In the meantime, however, there is no valid reason why we cannot compromise, as Dr. Hayward has suggested, and "translate the good things of home delivery to the hospital."

When a son is born at home, the question may arise about when and where he is to be circumcised. All Jewish babies are circumcised, and circumcision is now almost routine in American hospital births.

There is some evidence that the incidence of cervical cancer is

Family-Centered Maternity Care 243

considerably lower among Jewish women than among women in backward countries, where circumcision is not often performed. There is often a lack of personal cleanliness among such people, so that the natural secretion, *smegma*, collects under the foreskin and is not washed away before coitus. Bacteria and other infectious matter may have collected in the *smegma* and be deposited in the woman's body during intercourse. (The Old Testament patriarchs might have been surprised to find that this ritual procedure also provided a safeguard for his wife's health!)

The Old Testament suggests that circumcision be performed on the eighth day after birth (Lev. 12:3). There is a good medical reason for this. The substance in the blood necessary for coagulation (prothrombin) decreases in all infants during the first days of life, and the lack of this substance is most pronounced on the second to fifth day. It usually rises again spontaneously between the seventh and the tenth day, so that there is less bleeding, and healing occurs more rapidly if the circumcision is performed at that time.

The baby can be taken to the hospital as an outpatient for the circumcision, if it is to be performed. However, the New Testament indicates that circumcision is not mandatory (I Cor. 7:18, 19). An uncircumcised boy should be taught how to keep himself clean as he grows older.

THE PROPPED POSITION FOR BIRTH

One of the best things about having a baby at home rather than in the hospital is that it is possible to get into a comfortable, efficient position for bearing down properly in the second stage of labor. Primitive women use a variety of postures for giving birth to their babies, but almost always they have something to brace their feet against, and they draw their knees up toward their chests and bend their heads forward. This helps to relax the pelvic floor, widens the bony outlet, and aids the muscles of expulsion. In more highly developed cultures, the "birthstool" came into use. This enabled mothers to assume the same effective "bearing down" position, and among some groups it was used until the last century.

Dr. Michael Newton, chief of the Department of Obstetrics and Gynecology at the University of Mississippi, tells of the advantages of such a position, which can be made possible by means of a back rest:

> Use of the back rest has indicated that it has advantages for both obstetrician and patient. . . . For the obstetrician, the position is compatible with modern obstetrical practice. Satisfactory asepsis and control of delivery can be maintained. The back rest can easily be lowered if necessary. Intermittent general or regional anesthesia can be used. It is easier to work with a cooperative patient. . . . For the patient, the propped position enables her to take a more active and positive part in delivery. In a study done at the University of Mississippi Hospital comparing 217 women delivered in the propped position with 132 women delivered in the conventional lithotomy position, it was found that women who were propped were able to push better in the second stage, required less anesthesia and were more cooperative and had shorter third stages of labor when propped. Primiparas were more likely to be pleased at the first sight of their babies. . . . Patients themselves found the propped position more comfortable and satisfactory.[11]

In addition to being propped up, it is also essential to be able to move the legs freely from a pushing to a resting position between contractions. This is possible in a home birth but not in the hospital, where nothing is provided to brace one's feet against and where the legs are often strapped down. When one's legs are pinned down into a rigid, unchanging position, aching or cramping occurs, and circulation is impaired.

Is it possible to "translate the good things" of a comfortable effective, propped position, easily used in a home birth, to a hospital situation? The answer is yes.

Adjustable obstetric back rests are now available from several companies that manufacture delivery tables. In the absence of a suitable back rest, an inverted straight-backed chair on the delivery table makes a fine substitute, with the mother leaning against the chair legs, which are covered with pillows.

A homemade back rest can be made for a few dollars by any

husband handy with tools. It can be made to fit the bed or delivery table on which it is to be used. Instructions are in Appendix B.

Even with a back rest, it is helpful for the husband to help support his wife as she leans forward in bearing down.

ROOMING-IN

Another advantage of a home birth is the constant presence of one's baby and the opportunities this provides for frequent skin-to-skin contact between mother and infant, so important to an infant's healthy development. A dressed baby brought to the mother from the nursery, even for breast feeding, does not provide the same opportunity for skin-to-skin contact. The mother needs to handle and fondle her baby from head to toe, holding him close to her own bare arms and breast, dressing and undressing him with her own hands. This establishes a mutual closeness and sense of security from the very beginning.[12] Pediatricians are becoming aware of the symptoms of mental illness in small babies who are deprived of their mothers. Dr. Harry Bakwin writes:

> Infants under 6 months of age who have been in an institution for some time present a well-defined picture. The outstanding features are listlessness, emaciation and pallor, relative immobility, quietness, unresponsiveness to stimuli like a smile or a coo, indifferent appetite, failure to gain weight properly despite the ingestion of diets which, in the home, are entirely adequate, frequent stools, poor sleep, an appearance of unhappiness, proneness to febrile episodes, absence of sucking habits.[13]

Florence Blake, an associate professor in the nursing care of children at the University of Chicago, says there are infants in nearly every central nursery for the newborn who show some evidence of maternal deprivation. This is not surprising when one also learns that in the average nursery, each infant cries an average of 113.2 minutes a day—almost two hours.

> Although care in the nursery where the observations were made was excellent as judged by current standards, one would

question the nursing care on any floor where the average adult patient found it necessary to ring the service bell two hours out of every day.[14]

No one can measure the emotional trauma inflicted upon a tiny baby whose needs are not met. By contrast, rooming-in wards are quiet. Niles Newton says of one rooming-in ward she visited, that "there was almost a church-like hush as each mother nursed, or rocked, or slept with or near her own baby."[15]

Those of us who have mothered several children know that this kind of coddling of a tiny infant does not lead to spoiled, demanding babies. On the contrary, they become contented, happy, quickly responsive to affection. When this loving attention is given right from birth, we have not had the exhausting task of caring for a fussy baby who has developed the habit of long and frequent crying spells during his first four or five days in a central nursery. It takes us days, or weeks, to break this frustrated crying habit and to restore contentment to our tiny child when this has occurred.

Not only does the child need the mother, but the mother also needs her child, Miss Blake reminds us:

Continuity in the mother-child relationship is essential for both the child and the personality growth of the mother. Thus far continuity of care has been emphasized as being important to the child. It is equally essential for the mother.[16]

Reva Rubin, associate professor of maternity nursing at the University of Pittsburgh, demonstrates how the narcissistic introspection of the pregnant mother carries over to include her newborn child:

[There is] the compulsive need to ascertain that the baby is whole and intact. . . . Some mothers sneak looks under the blankets if they are not permitted to unwrap the baby. . . . The mother sees the minutest blemish with anguish: milia, petechiae, lanugo, dry skin, et cetera. There is an intolerance for anything short of perfection. . . . Her desperate need for both bodily intactness and perfection in her infant serve mother and infant richly and poignantly in a specifically maternal way. . . .

During the first week, each of the normal functions is checked on by the mother. If he never cries, she is relieved to learn that he can cry. If he never opens his eyes when she sees him, she worries and fusses until he does open his eyes. If he never has a wet diaper or a soiled diaper, she is silent until she finds that he can wet, he can move his bowels. How much she worries about his capacity to function physically can be realized by her expression of relief in laughter or tears when she finds that this, too, is all right.[17]

This hidden anxiety is spared the mother who rooms-in with her baby. Her fears are quickly proven unjustified. In addition, if she is breast-feeding her baby, she will find that she and the child will adjust to a more satisfactory breast-feeding pattern before returning home.

Rooming-in has advantages for the father, too, as he is included in the closeness of the family unit. Miss Blake writes:

> The father needs recognition as an important part of the family unit. "Rooming-in" helps to fulfill this need and to make obstetric care a family affair. In the "rooming-in" units the father is welcome not only because his wife needs him but also because he, too, needs opportunities to make an adjustment to the changes that have occurred within his family. . . . The arrival of a new child makes additional demands upon him, and unless his needs are met he may become frustrated and resentful, and seek to meet his dependency needs in nonconstructive ways. . . . Participating in the care of his child helps many fathers to accept and become identified with him. . . . Through shared experiences of this kind, family relationships become strengthened, and the possibilities for happy home life are increased.[18]

There is an even more pragmatic reason why rooming-in is not only necessary but essential, and that is the high incidence of infections among infants in central nurseries for the newborn, no matter how careful the aseptic routine may be. Dr. Newton relates a graphic example of this:

> The superiority of compulsory rooming-in over all nursery control techniques was demonstrated in an epidemic in an 84 bed

community general hospital with 750 live births a year. Telephone surveys were used as a method of ascertaining the extent of the epidemic, since 65.9% of the infant lesions and 93.3% of the maternal lesions occurred after discharge. Measures instituted to control the epidemic were: (1) removal of hospital personnel who were nasal carriers of the 80/81 strain of staphylococcus from the hospital nursery; (2) improvement of aseptic technique; and (3) discharge of infants and mothers three days after delivery. When all these measures appeared futile and only after closure of the maternity unit was being seriously considered by the staff, was compulsory rooming-in tried. This stopped the epidemic. Whereas 37.5% of the infants were infected under nursery care, only 5.0% were infected after compulsory rooming-in care. Maternal infection decreased from 5.1% to 1.4% after rooming-in was instituted.[19]

Some doctors say that new mothers do not want rooming-in, because they want a "vacation" while they are in the hospital and that they "don't want to be bothered" with the care of their infants. One wonders why such women "bothered" to have babies at all.

It is true that a new mother needs rest, although the natural childbearing mother does not feel sick and so regains her strength more quickly than others. Even so, any satisfactory rooming-in arrangement must provide adequate provision for a mother to rest undisturbed when this is necessary, while nurses look after her infant.

The floor plan described earlier makes this provision. Hospitals with this arrangement have two-, three-, or four-bed maternity rooms on each side of a wide central hall. There are openings in the walls at intervals, each containing a sliding-drawer bassinet, so placed that the sleeping baby can be drawn in beside the mother's bed at a touch. Nurses can tell by glancing down the central hall which babies are in their semiprivate nurseries and which babies are with their mothers.

This arrangement makes it possible for a mother to have her baby with her as much, or as little, as she likes. It enables her to sleep peacefully, knowing that her infant will still be under constant observation. It relieves nurses of the time wasted in carrying babies back and forth from a central nursery at feeding time. The Kaiser Memorial Hospital in Los Angeles is one that effectively uses the sliding-drawer bassinets in its rooming-in plan.

In addition, each mother should have toilet, wash basin, and shower facilities easily accessible. A central dining hall should be provided for the new mothers, and a lounge or sun porch where they can visit, so that each one can be up and out of bed as much as she likes. One reason a mother's strength returns so much more quickly after a home birth is that she can be up and about the house as much as she wants. Lying in bed most of the time for three to six days makes anyone feel weaker, not stronger. But in the hospital, if there is no place to go, a mother will spend too much time in bed. It gets a little boring just pacing up and down the halls.

One wonders how it is possible for any intelligent person to question the necessity and validity of rooming-in at all. Dr. Herbert Ratner describes its advantages with a touch of humor:

> We have now recently brought into the hospital nursery— that efficiently conducted displaced-persons concentration camp —a mechanical heart-beat to substitute for the reassuring heart-beat the baby would normally hear when at its mother's bosom. It is called the Securatone—shades of Wells, Huxley, and Orwell!
>
> Recent monkey experiments suggest that we should add to these automatic contrivances a heated, soft, skin-simulating latex covering. Within this mommy dummy, the Securatone, like a musical box in a doll, could perhaps be inserted appropriately. . . . It would seem that somewhere along the line some bright pediatrician might exclaim, "Eureka! Why don't we use the mother?"[20]

Dr. Robert A. Bradley suggests that the best plan of all is to send mother and baby home a couple of hours after a natural birth. This plan provides an excellent compromise for the hospital versus home birth question, and it also takes advantage of the physical exhilaration and exuberance one feels after a natural birth. As this excitement subsides, where can one rest more completely and happily, than at home in one's own bed? This doctor writes:

Healthy mothers, capable and eager to walk from the delivery room with their husbands at their sides and babies in their arms can see no reason for being "hospitalized" after giving birth. They repeatedly point out they are not *sick!*

We feel the benefits of "rooming-in" are multiple and justifiable, but the expense prohibitive. Our patients are instructed to have the assistance of another woman at home for the first two weeks to help with the household chores. They are told they must stay in the hospital two hours after the birth (the fourth stage of labor), but in the absence of complications or medications, may go home whenever they wish.

An added factor of safety is the reduction of postpartum hemorrhage by immediate breast feeding in 85 per cent of our mothers. This is primarily possible due to the activity of seven local chapters of the "La Leche League," wherein both husband and wife have received prenatal instruction in their roles relative to breast feeding. They are further reassured of continuous availability of advice during the postpartum by experienced officers of this nationwide organization.

This not only releases many hospital beds for others, but adds the psychological benefits of home environment, demand feeding, and "T. L. C." of the infant, and reduction of cross infections of baby and mother from exposure to others.

As Dr. Thaddeus L. Montgomery has stressed, "The hospital is a good place to deliver a baby but a poor place to board it."[21]

NURSE-MIDWIFERY

Until recently, almost all women were traditionally delivered by other women. By physical and emotional endowment women are particularly well suited for this task. But the traditional "midwife," while she gave the mother warm understanding and encouragement, too often lacked sufficient medical knowledge to protect both mother and child.

In other countries this problem has been solved by giving the midwife a professional, specialized training, and continuing to use her, but in the United States, unfortunately, she has had her task almost completely taken over by doctors.

But there are not enough doctors today to provide adequate maternity care. Among the nonwhite population, 83 per cent of whom are now being delivered by doctors in hospitals, a large percentage of premature infants are born because the mothers have had little or no prenatal care or training. Even the majority of the white population, who can afford the finest medical care, do not receive sufficient help during either pregnancy or labor.

The reason is not because our doctors are not capable but primarily because they do not have time to conduct prenatal classes, nor time to spend discussing with each pregnant patient her hopes and fears. Their management of her labor and birth is often restricted to a few momentary physical appraisals of the progress of her labor, returning to help her again only in time to "catch the baby." This state of affairs troubles many doctors as much as it does the patients. They would like to give more emotional support to each woman, but they are so rushed as it is that they have no time for themselves, no time for study or reflection, no time for their families.

The only adequate, permanent solution to this dilemma is to train many thousands more women for nurse-midwifery, in order to ease the doctors' burden and to provide more satisfying maternity care. The nurse-midwife receives much more training than the average maternity nurse working in hospitals. She not only receives a nurse's education, but takes additional graduate work in obstetrics. Few people understand how much education is involved. Delores Henne, who took her nurse-midwifery training at the Maternity Center in New York, said during her experience:

> During the past months, I have been asked frequently, "What are you doing?" I reply, "I am taking a course in nurse-midwifery." In turn, I hear interesting comments such as: "I thought midwifery went out of the window when horses and buggies went out." Few seem to know that nurse-midwifery is a postgraduate course for registered nurses, training them to give the normal pregnant mother antenatal care, deliver her baby, and post-partal care.[22]

Dr. Nicholson Eastman of the University of Minnesota School of Medicine reports that after observing one nurse-midwife program in which these women delivered over six hundred babies, he is convinced of the need for many more nurse-midwives:

> In this entire experience, these young women have not made a single serious mistake, that is, a mistake which endangered the life of mother or child. . . . In the Prenatal Clinic, they take time to answer in detail the patient's puzzlements and in labor they never leave her. They are quick to spot the abnormal and quick to transfer such abnormalities to the obstetricians; and in the remaining perfectly normal cases they provide a type of maternity care which is superior.[23]

Courses in nurse-midwifery are now being conducted by the Maternity Center Association of New York City, in conjunction with the Kings County Hospital, the State University of New York, and the Columbia-Presbyterian Medical Center. Other courses are conducted at Yale University, the Johns Hopkins Hospital, the Catholic Maternity Institute in New Mexico (affiliated with the Catholic University), the Frontier Graduate School of Midwifery in Hyden, Kentucky, and the University of Puerto Rico.

The Maternity Center Association in New York has graduates in nurse-midwifery now working in twenty-six other countries, because they have not been well accepted in the United States. For this reason, we have only five hundred nurse-midwives. In England, by contrast, there are *fifteen thousand* practicing nurse-midwives. These nurse-midwives lose fewer babies per thousand births than American doctors, and the nurse-midwives of Sweden, who deliver 85 per cent of the babies there, lose just a little over half as many babies per thousand births as we do.

In comparison with Russia, our lack of adequate personnel for maternity care is startling. The *Report of the Medical Exchange Mission to the USSR, Maternal and Child Care,*[24] states that Russia now has eighteen physicians per ten thousand population, while the United States has only 13.2 physicians per ten thousand population. Russia is graduating new physicians (six years of medical school) at the rate of twenty thousand a year, while the United States is graduating only 6,861 a year, not nearly enough even to maintain the present ratio of 13.2 per ten thousand population. And *in addition,* Russia has 200,000 excellently trained midwives.

The Russians place priority on maternal and child health, as has been mentioned before. Every pregnant woman, in cities or rural areas, receives prenatal examinations monthly (and more often the last two months) by an obstetrician. She also receives six lessons in natural childbirth and six lessons in the care of the infant.

Ordinarily, one Russian midwife is assigned to every two women and stays with them throughout labor and birth. An obstetrician is always available if there are complications, or a need for manipulation or forceps delivery.

In the maternity section, one nurse is assigned to every three or four women, and one to every two newborn. For premature babies, one medical attendant is assigned to each infant. "The delegation was impressed by the abundance of personnel."

The main drawback in Russian obstetrics is the mechanistic attitude. Giving birth is a "science." Husbands are not included, and there is no family-centered maternity care. But, in spite of this serious omission, these facts underline the desperate need in the United States for more nurse-midwifery schools and for many thousands more young women to enter this most worthwhile profession. Nurse-midwives can help to correct the widespread criticism of our present hospital "assembly-line," "impersonal" care of the woman in labor. They have been the ones most active and vocal in helping those of us who are anxious for more homelike circumstances in hospital deliveries.

The Catholic sisters are providing especially fine leadership in family-centered maternity care programs in hospitals, such as the one at St. Mary's Hospital in Evansville, Indiana, under the direction of Sister Mary Stella Simpson, past president of the American College of Nurse-Midwives.

It is to be hoped that many of our Protestant hospitals will also begin to provide the needed leadership in establishing family-centered maternity care. There is emphasis in these hospitals on the need for meeting the needs of the "whole" man—his spiritual as well as his physical needs, but this emphasis is not applied to the labor and maternity units. Too often there is no emphasis on maintaining the integrity of the family unit during childbirth and the puerperium and no realization that this, too, is an area in which the hospital has an obligation in its spiritual ministry.

For the young woman looking forward to an area of service one can think of few more needed and rewarding areas for her to minister, than nurse-midwifery. As a matter of fact, this is a service in which women who have raised a family could contribute a great deal. Those who have had nurses' training could take time out to review their training and take special training in nurse-midwifery. Older women are especially suited for this task, having been taught patience and understanding during the years of coping with the tantrums and trials of the two-year-olds and the teens. In many cultures a woman must have reared a family to enter the honorable calling of midwifery. But whether young or middle-aged, the American nurse-midwife—though much better trained—can approach her responsibilities with the same sense of dedication as the old granny midwives of the South, who claimed that "granny midwives always been called by the Lord, like preachers are."[25]

These granny midwives took their calling as a spiritual service to God, and their personal self-sacrifice and devotion to duty remains a challenge to anyone working in obstetrics. One old soul at the time of her retirement said, "I been passing faithful and never quit till the Lord knowed I can't hardly get along, and He lifted all the burden He laid on me." Another one said:

> I caught a lots of babies when their mothers birthed them. . . . Over forty years I been a granny midwife and no mother ever died with me. But I don't take credit to myself. I always had the Lord and one or the other Doc Powells to call on in trouble. . . .

> Now I'm old and bent over and sometimes when I get called in the nighttime, I says, "Lord, I'm old and tired. Give me my long rest and let me come up there to stay." . . . But the Lord He says, "You ain't so old as you will be. I got work yet for you to do down there and I'll give you strength. Go long now, and do your job!"[26]

Notes

1. Dale Clark, "A Man's Crusade for Easy Childbirth," *Esquire,* October 1949.
2. Robert A. Bradley, M.D., "The Role of the Husband in Natural Childbirth," *1960 ICEA Convention Report,* pp. 68, 69. Reprinted by permission.
3. Ernestine Wiedenbach, *Family-Centered Maternity Nursing* (New York: G. P. Putnam's Sons, 1958).
4. Robert A. Bradley, M.D., "Fathers' Presence in Delivery Rooms," *Psychosomatics,* Vol. III, No. 6, November–December 1962, p. 5. Reprinted by permission.
5. Bernard Eaton, "Should a Father See His Baby Born?" *The American Weekly,* January 15, 1956.
6. Mrs. Walter Bowman, "Story of a Natural Childbirth," *Child-Family Digest,* January 1955, p. 101. Reprinted by permission.
7. Delores Henne, R.N., C.N.M., in a letter to Mrs. T. D. Lutz for the column "We the Women," *The Baptist Herald* (Forest Park, Ill.: North American Baptist General Conference), January 24, 1957, p. 16. Reprinted by permission.
8. Gillian Mitchell, nurse-midwife, in the panel discussion "Approaches to Childbirth Around the World," printed in the *ICEA 1962 Convention Report,* pp. 5, 6. Reprinted by permission.
9. Herbert Thom, M.D., *Childbirth—With Understanding* (Springfield, Ill.: C. Thomas, 1962), p. 83. Reprinted by permission.
10. Ashley Montagu, Ph.D., "Should Babies Be Born at Home?" *The Humanization of Man* (New York: World Publishing Co., 1962), Chap. 8.
11. Michael Newton, M.D., "The Use of the Propped Position for Delivery," an unpublished paper. Reprinted by permission.
12. Ashley Montagu, *Touching, The Human Significance of the Skin* (New York: Columbia University Press, 1971).
13. Florence G. Blake, R.N., *The Child, His Parents and the Nurse* (Philadelphia: Lippincott, 1954), p. 6, quoting Harry Bakwin, "Emotional Deprivation in Infants," *Journal of Pediatrics,* 1949, Vol. 35, p. 512. Reprinted by permission.
14. Niles Newton, Ph.D., "The Medical Case for Routine Rooming-In," *Child and Family,* January 1962. Reprinted by permission.
15. *Ibid.*
16. Blake, *The Child, His Parents and the Nurse,* p. 10. Reprinted by permission.

17. Reva Rubin, R.N., C.N.M., "Basic Maternal Behavior," *Nursing Outlook*, November 1961, pp. 684–86. Reprinted by permission.
18. Blake, *The Child, His Parents and the Nurse*, p. 79. Reprinted by permission.
19. Newton, "The Medical Case for Routine Rooming-In." Reprinted by permission.
20. Herbert Ratner, M.D., "Medicine" (Santa Barbara Center for the Study of Democratic Institutions), p. 38. Reprinted by permission.
21. Bradley, "Fathers' Presence in Delivery Rooms." Reprinted by permission.
22. Henne, letter to Mrs. Lutz. Reprinted by permission.
23. Thoms, *Childbirth—With Understanding*, p. 71. Reprinted by permission.
24. *Report of the Medical Exchange Mission to the USSR*, Public Health Service Publication No. 954, pp. 1, 4, 18, 35.
25. Marie Campbell, *Folks Do Get Born* (New York: Rinehart and Co., 1946), p. 109. This book is a delightful tale of the personalities of the Negro midwives who worked under the direction of the Public Health nurses in Georgia.
25. *Ibid.*

Chapter 21

Natural Childbirth

A HUMANITARIAN PHILOSOPHY

One of the main tenets of natural childbirth is that every pregnant and parturient woman must be cared for on an individual basis, according to her individual physical and emotional needs and desires. A woman longs to remain a *person* throughout her childbearing experience. When a young wife, pregnant for the first time, enters a doctor's office, does he attempt to know *her,* or does he immediately brush aside her feelings of youthful modesty and conduct a thorough physical examination? Is he unaware that she is not yet emotionally prepared for such an invasion of her spirit? We have all seen these young women, leaving the office blushing and subdued.

> When, therefore, the young married woman enters the consulting room believing, hoping or fearing that she is going to have a baby, the physician's first investigations should be to confirm that she is pregnant. This may be ascertained by clinical signs, without an internal or vaginal examination. Such an examination can be a severe shock to many young women and, apart from the discomfort it may cause, it is an experience that frequently produces a lack of confidence in the attendants. If at thirteen weeks the uterus is not in the correct place and position, a vaginal investigation should be carefully performed for sound clinical reasons.[1]

Such thoughtful consideration for preserving the integrity of her

257

innermost needs as a person helps a young woman to confide in her doctor. She becomes more responsive to his guidance toward a rewarding birth experience. She realizes that he does not regard her simply as a reproductive machine, to be prodded and examined, doped and delivered when her time comes.

Thorough training in the principles of natural childbirth and how to achieve it is the right of every pregnant woman. But because each woman is an individual, not all will respond favorably to such teaching. The doctor who is aware of the emotional needs of his patient will courteously comply with her wishes to be "knocked out" to the extent that he considers it safe to do so. Dr. Dick-Read was the first to write:

> . . . a serious word of warning—no one who uses these methods must expect invariable success. There are women who will never learn control, who will never concentrate upon doing their antenatal work well, and whose upbringing has given them a psychological background upon which fear thrives. Analgesics and anesthetics are the correct treatment for such. Whatever happens, no woman should ever be allowed to persist in pain.[2]

Such women are in the minority, however. There are also a few women who have physical abnormalities that necessitate anesthetics. But the majority of young women respond eagerly to adequate childbirth training and are profoundly grateful afterward for the guidance they received. In their happy natural birth experiences they have come face to face for the first time with the real meaning of being *woman,* and they have found it good.

> . . . The experience of normal labor and nursing are important steps in a young woman's personality growth, character development and emotional adulthood and . . . successful accomplishment of these acts helps to release her from childhood feelings of inadequacy and need for dependence on others. Many stable women have an intuitive understanding of this point. . . . The violent opposition expressed by others is a defensive mechanism through which they justify their subconscious rejection of submerged feelings of inadequacy and passive dependence.[3]

The average doctor does not seem to understand this intuitive need for fulfillment in the childbearing experience that a young woman feels. What he does not understand, he does not approve. When he does not approve, he is unwilling to help her to achieve her goal. When he is unwilling to help her, he is failing in his responsibilities to her as her physician. Fortunately, situations like this are on the decline, as the late Dr. M. Leonard Kimmel illustrated in June 1962 when he said:

> I must say that education for childbirth has been increasing through the years. . . . It's coming along very rapidly. Even though I was the only doctor among 640 in my county to practice natural childbirth, I don't think there's an obstetrician on the staff of my hospital, who has not had at least one case of "so-called' natural childbirth. Some women wanted to and were like Julie Harris—strong enough to fight the anesthetist, and the doctors were "good" enough to let them go through with it. Having done one, now they're waiting for others. I don't believe a woman should have to fight the anesthetist.[4]

THE MIRACLE OF BIRTH

1. *The first stage of labor.*

Civilization has imposed one handicap upon us that primitive women did not have to contend with. Women have to puzzle over whether labor has or has not begun, in order to know whether to go or not to go to the hospital. In the majority of women the beginning of true labor is signaled by contractions that occur at regular intervals. But for some this is not an infallible sign of true labor. Contractions are occurring every three and a half minutes. She is told to report to the hospital. She packs her bag and goes. Several hours later she is dismissed, the regular contractions having ceased. She is told that she was in "false" labor.

Then again, a woman thinks she is in labor. She calls the doctor. "Are the contractions regular?" he asks, and she replies that they are not. She is told to call again as soon as they become regular. An hour later the parents and doctor rush to the hospital, and the baby appears shortly. Her contractions never did become regular.

For those who have this difficulty, how is it possible to know whether labor is "true" or "false"? A safer criterion is especially necessary for the mother who has learned to relax, as some contractions may pass unnoticed, and she will not think they are "regular."

Because this may be a problem, certain sensations that are true indications of labor should be recognized. The surest way to tell if the contractions are real or "practice" ones, is by noticing whether or not there is this mild feeling of tightening *down in the area of the pubic bone and lower spine.* This is a sign that the uterine muscles are pushing *down.* A false contraction will often be much larger, expanding the abdomen up and out, rather than giving this sensation of tightening *low* in the abdomen. This sensation disappears when one relaxes, so *do not go to bed* to relax if you think that you are really in labor. Wait to relax completely until you are in the hospital.

Once in the hospital, consciously allowing all muscles of the abdomen and pelvic area to be limply relaxed, many contractions may pass unnoticed. One mother tells of it in this way:

> One strange thing occurred that puzzled me. From time to time, the nurse would put her hand on my abdomen and say, "Are you having a contraction?" And in all truth I would answer, "I don't think so, I don't feel anything." "Well, you are," she would answer, "only you must be so relaxed that you don't feel it."[5]

Medical attendants in the labor wards should realize how much pain they cause indirectly by their constant concern over the strength and regularity of labor contractions. "Be sure to tell the nurses when your *pains* get too bad," the doctor says kindly. Or, "Oh, that's a *good* one," the nurse at our side remarks, her hand on our rising abdomen. She stands expectantly, watch in hand, waiting for the next one. Unconsciously we begin to tense in anticipation of the "next one" along with her, embarrassed at keeping her waiting when she is so patient. All this preoccupation with contractions contributes to pain. As one obstetrician aptly said, "If we paid this much attention to the processes of digestion, we'd all have nervous in-digestion!" Another eminent doctor reminds us of this:

> Our organs actually work much better when we leave them to their automatic functioning and do not think about them. That this is so is clearly shown in the case of the hypochondriac, who suffers from all kinds of functional disorders simply because his mind occupies itself with his body. These disorders attract the attention of his mind, and thus he is caught in a vicious circle.[6]

When in the hospital in labor, one must rest quietly, ignoring the contractions during the first stage of labor. If they begin to cause discomfort, it helps to change to the left lateral position, with a pillow under one's upper knee. It is *most* important for the right knee and thigh to be supported, so that the abdomen sags loosely toward the bed, while the upper leg and knee support one's weight. Sometimes a mild sedative is given if one has difficulty in relaxing:

> If tension-pain-cycle continues so that there is resistance to several successive contractions, a small dose of medication, e.g., Demerol 50 mg. or Pethedine 50 mg., can help the mother to relax again and co-operate with the forces of labour. Large doses of analgesics or sedatives tend to make it difficult to co-operate effectively and can be unsafe for baby.[7]

It is impossible to remain in one position for long periods of time. For those who seem unable to get comfortable in the lateral position and prefer to lie in the reclining-chair position, their back and knees must be elevated and supported to prevent tension on the abdominal muscles. Sometimes the labor-room bed is too narrow for lying in the lateral position. In this case, a mother can lie on her side with a large pillow between her knees. This will hold them apart, keep the weight of the upper leg from resting on the lower one, and help her keep the pelvic floor relaxed.

As transition approaches, it may become necassary to concentrate on controlled breathing to stay relaxed. It is most important, however, for attendants to remember that the woman before them is an *individual*. Some have been trained in slightly different procedures for attaining a natural birth from the ones familiar to the nurse. Marjorie Karmel, who learned the psychoprophylactic procedure for avoiding pain, describes the rude way attendants treated her in an American hospital:

> The contractions had become very strong. I was quite cantankerous about making nurses wait till they were over to listen to the foetal heartbeat. Then a new nurse wandered in to take her crack at me. She had short red hair and a delicate twinkle in her eye. Seeing that I was doing some sort of activity of my own, she stood by the bed and waited until the contraction in progress was over. "Well," she said to Alex. "Just look at that! She seems to have worked out a little system all her own. She's patting her tummy and panting like a puppy. Look," she added to Dr. Sedley who had just come in. "She's patting her tummy and panting like a puppy, and it seems to do her good!"[8]

Mrs. Karmel was using the controlled breathing and abdominal massage she had learned in France. Because it was new to her attendants, it was scoffed at. One can share her indignation!

2. *The transition period.*

There are certain emotional signs of the progress of labor that a woman shows. These make it possible for attendants to tell how her labor is advancing without frequent rectal examinations, which always interfere with relaxation. By observing these phenomena, both mother and attendants can tell when the transition period is near. Dr. Virginia Larsen writes:

> The inexperience of the hospital team with trained parents may make them under-evaluate the shortened labors and the woman's self-awareness of labor progress; consequently the obstetrician is apt to be called too late. Many nurses are not aware of the emotional pattern of labor and miss the importance of the signs of the transition period from the first to the second stage. As the emotional guideposts in labor become more appreciated, the labor room nurse, and the intern will find these a valuable adjunct to the rectal exams that otherwise tend to be overdone and discomforting.[9]

These emotional guideposts have been outlined as follows: The mother appears mildly euphoric and frequently likes to carry on conversation between contractions until the cervix is dilated to about four centimeters; at three to four centimeters she becomes more serious about her labor; as transition approaches, the mother may find difficulty in relaxing, experience some backache, and she may also feel chilled to the point where her legs will tremble. When this happens, the attendants will probably wrap her warmly in blankets and give her a hot water bottle and have her change to the reclining-chair position on the bed.

Transition contractions usually last a full minute or more, and they may come so close together that they seem almost continuous. This is the point in labor when an uninstructed woman may go all to pieces emotionally and remain out of control for the rest of the time. *No woman should ever be left alone after labor has begun.*

During transition (eight to ten centimeters until complete dilation) there is often a feeling of confusion between the need to *relax*, as for first-stage contractions, and the need to *push*, as for second-stage contractions. The mother should be reminded not to bear down until the doctor gives his permission, since pushing too soon can damage the cervix. It helps to be raised to a sitting position during transition, with the knees raised and supported by pillows or the stirrups, so the legs can remain limp.

The strength of transition contractions may alarm a woman having her first baby. If she has had a relaxed, comfortable first stage, the sensation of the strong contractions will be similar to that of tensing her biceps firmly in the upper arm. She should be reminded that transition is very short and that she will soon be more comfortable.

As the transition stage ends, the bearing-down reflex begins. This reflex may not begin immediately after the cervix is completely dilated; the uterine muscles need time to shorten, since the baby is now farther down. If pushing causes any discomfort, the mother should be told to wait and not push until it does not hurt. If her body is ready, bearing down will feel good.

3. *The birth of the baby.*

The second stage of labor is the really exciting period. At last one can *do* something to help bring this baby into the world! Inhalant anesthetics should be available if they are needed, but many share the sentiments of the mother who wrote:

> Then into the delivery room, and they said, "Here, take this." "No!" . . . About four times they offered it and I refused. Why they offer it, I'll never know. Tell your girls if they can get out of the labor room without anesthetic, whatever they do, don't take any in the delivery room. They've had *all the pain* they'll have in the whole process already, and by taking gas they'll cheat themselves of the most fascinating, thrilling series of sensations they've ever experienced![10]

Frequently a young mother needs to be reminded not to "squeeze up" the muscles of her pelvic floor as she feels the baby's head coming down, but to keep them slack. Often she will hesitate to relax this birth outlet and bear down properly because of shyness and embarrassment over this part of her body. Turning her attention to her baby as soon as possible helps to relieve her self-consciousness and relax the outlet by taking her mind off herself. If the muscles of the outlet remain tense, she will have pain.

A common mistake that is made is instructing the woman to bear down "as if moving the bowels." This increases her embarrassment and is confusing. This advice causes the woman to tighten the vagina in order to open the anus. This hinders, rather than helps, her efforts.

As the baby's head descends and the initial stretching of the vulva begins, the mother may appear alarmed. Although this "pins and needles" sensation is only mildly uncomfortable, it brings all the negative influences of our culture to mind. The common belief that the approaching moment of birth *will* be painful causes the mother to hesitate with doubt at this crucial point.

It is a wise attendant who can reassure her with confidence that the birth outlet will be insensitive in a moment, and that she will feel only the bulging of the baby's head. She will be grateful to him after the birth is over, if he does not rob her of the wonderful orgasm of birth by administering an anesthetic, or pudendal block,* or hypnotic analgesia, against her wishes.

One cannot feel either the incision for an episiotomy, or minor laceration during the birth, once the baby's head has cut off circulation of the blood to the perineum. What one *does* feel is the thrilling expansion of the vagina to its maximum capacity.

Mrs. Dick-Read describes a properly conducted delivery as follows:

> As the head is about to be born, the attendant will place a hand firmly on the area between the anus and the birth canal (perineum) supporting the head towards the mother as it emerges. . . . She will feel no pain as the head is born (contrary to popular belief) because nature provides a perfect numbing, for a few minutes, of the area surrounding the outlet. During the crowning and birth the mother can think of herself as "a rose unfolding" bringing her baby forth gently and beautifully as it should be.

> Irrespective of whether the attendant is present or not, the oncoming *head should never be held back forcibly* but should be allowed to be born slowly and gently. Nor should the baby be pulled straight out from the mother. The natural rotation of the head should be allowed to take place without interference, and the baby allowed to come gently of its own accord, supported *upwards* towards the mother's abdomen.

> . . . there is no immediate need to cut the cord which attaches the baby to its placenta. . . . [Wait until] pulsation has ceased.[11]

The description Dr. Dick-Read gives of his delivery of a child is vastly different from orthodox deliveries in America:

> . . . the mother will be holding the hands of the child before the body is born. The head emerges and with the next contraction the shoulders are freed. The child is then rotated and lies upward facing his mother. That rotation gives relief and takes the tension from the points where it has been greatest on the perineum. It is then we see an astonishing transfiguration of a hard-working woman employing the effort syndrome, which made her appear

---

* The pudendal block is administered by injecting an anesthetic into the mother's bottom with a huge needle. It deadens all of the immediate pelvic area, but not as large an area as the saddle block.

distressed, to a mother who suddenly becomes happy and smiling and sits up and waits for the baby to be fully born. Women in these circumstances will complain because the doctor is not yet able to tell them whether it is a boy or a girl. They will ask him to hurry, and I have to say to them, "I will hurry when you give me a contraction to hurry with."

. . . These children are all handed to the mother immediately after the cord is cut. Every woman takes her child in her arms and holds it to her breast, not necessarily to suckle it. This stimulates a reflex contraction of the uterus which is definitely of physiological value. I think women were meant to take their babies when born. They will say what a funny looking thing it is. "Is that the right colour, doctor?" "It really is like my husband!"[12]

4. *The delivery of the placenta.*

Mrs. Dick-Read describes the proper delivery of an afterbirth, which every mother should know and understand:

> The close contact between mother and child and the suckling of the child at the breast will cause the uterus to contract strongly, thus preventing excessive bleeding. There need be no hurry and there will be little maternal loss (bleeding) provided there is no pummelling or squeezing of the uterus.
>
> Any violent form of extrusion of the placenta is a violation of the purely natural function and has no place in a normal delivery. One should never attempt to hurry the birth of the placenta by impatient pulling on the cord. A sharp cough will usually jog the placenta and bring it forth if it is ready to come. . . . Injections to hurry the placenta and to prevent bleeding should only be given if there are clinical indications. There is very little loss of maternal blood after a carefully managed labour. . . . Once the placenta is delivered and the mother is refreshed there is no reason why she may not walk immediately if she wishes to do so.[13]

If a slight abrasion occurred during the birth, doctors who understand natural childbirth take the stitches immediately, while the perineum is still insensitive. It is only later, after the delivery of the afterbirth, that they are tied. This tying, if not carefully done, can cause more discomfort than the stitches, since feeling has by then returned to the perineum.*

The birth is not completed until the afterbirth has come. None of us can fully appreciate the miracle that has taken place within this simple organ. Dr. Dick-Read often uses this occasion to point his patient to God's part in the creation of a child:

> Years ago it was unheard of that a woman should wish to see the afterbirth. Today nearly every woman who watches her baby born asks me to show her the placenta. This I do, and point out the bag in which the infant, now lying peacefully in her arms, developed and became a perfect little human being. . . . "Madam, when man can make one of these, he will have reached the foot-stool of the Creator; as I hold this discarded mass in my hand, I am humbled by the limitations of Science."[14]

Having given birth without an anesthetic, it is astonishing how exuberant and energetic the mother feels right afterward. Mild activity, as well as rest, helps all body functions return to normal. Breast-feeding the baby a few moments from time to time aids the uterus in contracting. One can feel it knot into a hard ball as the baby takes the nipple. If he will not take the nipple into his mouth, help him to nuzzle it with his nose or cheek. This will have the same stimulating effect on the uterus.

5. *Breast-feeding the baby.*

The tiny baby needs much more than warmth and food. He also needs the kind of affection that the reassuring kinesthetic warmth of his mother's body gives him. Ashley Montagu suggests that a child's nine months in the womb may represent only half of his gestation period, the last half being completed after his birth, when he still needs the closeness of his mother's body.

Food is not simply nourishment; it is also an expression of love and friendship. Guests come to pay us a visit. We are glad to see them, and slip into the kitchen a bit later to prepare refreshments

---

* On the rare occasions when an episiotomy is necessary in a natural birth, some doctors use 1 or 2 per cent Novocain for the stitches if feeling has returned to the perineum.

for them. The obese person stuffs his body with food because he is starved for human affection and understanding. Our toddler falls and hurts himself. We comfort him with a cookie, and with a hug and kiss. In this same way we comfort him when he is tiny:

> The baby is put to the breast whenever he indicates discomfort. This feeding act helps to warm and soothe him. He may stay at the breast for a half hour or an hour at a time. The comfort he receives there encourages him to fuss for frequent repetition. The hours of sucking each day vigorously stimulate lactation. Milk in large quantities appears rapidly, often within 24 hours after birth.
>
> The baby and mother stay near each other through the first few months. Each night they sleep within touching distance, and in the daytime the baby is carried everywhere his mother goes. Feeding continues on demand day and night. The baby seldom cries for he is constantly within reach of the soothing comfort of his mother's breast, the warmness of her body, and the gentle touch of her skin.[15]

Thus breast-feeding gives the infant the security of love that he needs. Bottle feeding, theoretically, can do this, too, *if* we stop and hold our baby close each time he takes the bottle until he is several months old. But we do not do this. It is too easy, after the first few weeks, to pop a bottle in his mouth, prop it up on a pillow, and rush off to other pressing tasks. Our aims are high, but we do not fulfill them.

My own eighteen-month-old toddler occasionally showed this need for affection with his food. He was weaned from the breast but was too big to need to be held each time he took the bottle, which he still enjoyed. Occasionally he would not take it, no matter how hungry he was. He would pull me away from the sink, where I was washing dishes, or tug at my arm as I sat by the typewriter. He wanted more than food; he wanted *me*, his mother. So I would lay aside the urgent task at hand, hold him and rock him as he drank his milk. And then, his need for food and affection satisfied, he would play contentedly near me the rest of the morning as I went about my work.

Breast-feeding is as important for the mother as for the baby. It demands of her that she stop and relax frequently, which helps her to regain her strength more quickly. As she rocks and feeds her baby, or lies on the bed with him, she can doze, or read, or just enjoy admiring him. Breast-feeding is the most fun *after* the first three or four months, as the baby becomes more responsive. He stops drinking to smile at his mother, as if to say thank you. He pats the breast playfully with his little hands. He teases—now he will take the nipple in his mouth, now he will not, until she scolds him laughingly, "You naughty baby, get busy now!" This give-and-take relationship provides the mother with the security of love, too, which the child gives.

An additional advantage to breast-feeding for the mother, which few American women realize, is that it gives her a physical, as well as spiritual, sense of satisfaction and well-being. This is clearly explained in Niles Newton's article "The Sexual Implications of Breast Feeding":

> There is just as much physical basis for believing a woman should get pleasure from breast feeding as there is a physical basis for believing a woman should get pleasure from intercourse. Her nipples are extremely sensitive tissue which become erect when stimulated.
>
> Nipple stimulation, or psychic stimulation such as the baby's hunger cry, causes the discharge of a pituitary hormone which has the double effect of causing the uterus to contract rhythmically for as long as twenty minutes. . . .
>
> Undoubtedly, many frigid breast feeders exist. However, the existence of frigid breast feeders does not indicate that this condition is inevitable, any more than the existence of frigid males indicates that sexual frigidity is inevitable. Naturally, intercourse can involve more intense feelings; but breast feeding gives more frequent sensations. . . . As the infant grows older the frequency of breast feeding recedes. However, at the same time the child's sucking strength increases and the amount of milk discharged increases—thus increasing the physical pleasure possibilities of each nursing. . . .
>
> Successful breast feeding, as practiced by a large proportion

of peoples all over the world, is entirely different from the unsuccessful frigid breast feeding attempt by the modern urban American mother. Successful breast feeding is a simple and easy procedure. The hungry baby is merely lifted to the bared breast, and he and his mother join for a while in the lactation embrace. Doubt, worry, fear, and embarrassment are absent; and thus the mother is free to enjoy the physical sensations of the act. The mutual pleasure of the act is so satisfying that breast feeding often continues into the second or third year, or even longer.

It is indeed curious that the suggestion that women can and should get pleasure from sucking shocks many more than the suggestion that women can and should get pleasure from intercourse.[16]

Picture for a moment, some of the Renaissance paintings which captured the elusive beauty in the faces of mother and child, as they shared the physical and spiritual pleasures of the "lactation embrace." Can we imagine feeling the same moving response to a painting in which a mother is feeding her child with a bottle?

The great majority of mothers who have had a natural birth prefer to breast-feed their babies. Perhaps the common painful frigid birth experience forced on the American woman has inhibited her ability to breast-feed successfully and makes these attempts frigid also.

Mothers who live in areas where breast-feeding one's babies is not popular will find real encouragement from the mothers in La Leche League International (see Appendix A).

THE BIRTH CLIMAX

Because the birth climax is so important and yet so poorly understood, discussion of it has been left until now. The one thing that puzzles doctors most about natural childbirth is the enthusiasm of mothers who have experienced it to repeat it again and again and to pass on what we have learned to other women. One young mother, now a missionary in Japan, said to me, "People think that by 'painless' we mean that we don't *feel* anything. That's not true! We feel a great deal, but what we feel doesn't hurt."

Some doctors, realizing that we do "feel" something, have defined these pleasurable sensations as a sublimation of pain![17] People who feel pain as pleasure are masochistic or sadistic. They are not normal. Clearly, this explanation is inadequate.

The simple truth is that when a woman says, "It was such a thrill!" or, "I wouldn't have missed it for anything!" she is not just referring to the emotional excitement of being present when her child appeared but is also referring to a physical climax of her whole being that words simply can't describe.

The emotional excitement that accompanies the physical stimulation of the birth demands relief through expression. This results in a "crying out" similar to the involuntary gasp or cry as intercourse approaches the height of its climax. Too often this "crying out" is misinterpreted by attendants as a sign of pain!

An excellent example of this phenomenon is found in an early Russian novel, written by a woman, Lidiia Nikoloevna. The heroine, Verinea, is speaking:

> "I want my child to come into this world in joy. I have waited for it a long time. . . . I will not cry out, I wish it to have an easy birth." And she uttered a single cry, a loud, strong one. It did not seem to be a cry of pain, but one of joy. And then her body was pierced by an indescribably sweet, light sensation and she heard the marvellously lusty voice of the newborn child.

This "sweet, light sensation," which is similar to the release from the emotional impact at the height of orgasm in intercourse, is demonstrated in the dazed and happy expressions of a woman whose baby was born in a car on the way to the hospital recently:

> "Better get a doctor," she said calmly. . . . "The baby's here already." At this instant I heard it cry. It seemed incredible. . . . Dotty, *at peace,* lay against the seat . . . The attendant and I helped Dotty, who seemed *dazed and happy,* into a wheelchair. (Italics added.)[18]

The euphoric emotion that follows the birth climax subsides slowly, just as does a woman's excitement following the climax of intercourse, and the new mother should have companionship for a while after her child has been born naturally. She will relax and rest contentedly after this first happy wave of emotion has had time to subside.

This euphoria of newly delivered mothers is rarely witnessed by American doctors who try to apply the principles of natural childbirth, because most of them *insist on dulling the final climax, or birth orgasm,* as the baby emerges, by using a pudendal or saddle block, an inhalant anesthetic, or hypnotic analgesia and amnesia to deaden sensation in the pelvic area.

Fortunately, some doctors are now recognizing the similarity of a natural birth experience to a sexual experience. Dr. N. Kalichman, a graduate of McGill Medical School with postgraduate training at the Allen Memorial Institute of Psychiatry in Montreal, writes:

> An analogy drawn between childbirth and sexual intercourse sheds a new light on this idea. In labor, the descending baby can be considered the equivalent of the penis in intercourse. In both situations, the to and fro movements of the penis or baby accompany increasing intensity of stimuli received from the genitalia. A possible explanation now arises as to the mysterious dozing that occurs between contractions during the second stage, and of the amnesia experienced during a great part of the labor. These two phenomena are characteristic also for the period close to the climax of intercourse. A possible explanation for both situations in psychological terms presents itself. The ego withdraws from the too-intense stimulation into a semi-consciousness. . . . To continue the analogy, as the climax is reached in both situations, the woman utters involuntary sounds and performs involuntary pelvic movements. With the expulsion of the child, as in reaching the climax of the orgasm, the woman suddenly relaxes, and there appears a calm ecstatic look on her face. The analogy applies as well to the post-delivery state. The woman's remarks are now directed to both the child and physician and are usually tender and loving and are reminiscent of remarks following intercourse. . . . As in intercourse, the ideal may not be attained, and the expression of some of these various natural phenomena may be inhibited.[19]

The following delightfully uninhibited account of the birth of a child verifies Dr. Kalichman's observations. The mother who wrote it was twenty-four years old when her child was born. It was her first child, weighed 9 pounds, 12 ounces, and was 21 inches long. She titled her account, completed when her baby was ten days old, "I Want a Thousand Babies":

Doctor said. . . . "When you feel a contraction coming, pull." Doubtfully I tried pulling, and it seemed pleasant, but only that. Then, on the next contraction I started to pull, and was suddenly swept away with primitive strength. Everything went blank and lightninglike streaks flashed, it seemed. It was ecstatic, wonderful, thrilling! I . . . heard myself moaning—in triumph, not in pain! There was no pain whatsoever, only a primitive and sexual elation. From my grimace, the nurse thought I was in pain and started to put the mask over my face. How annoying! In the middle of a push, I gasped, "Go away! It doesn't hurt."

I felt as if I had enough strength to pull the world apart— everything was bright, illuminated. In between contractions, I shouted deliriously, *"This is wonderful!* My husband only wants two babies, but I want a thousand." . . . And then another contraction started. The doctor said, "I know it feels good to shout, but don't do it; that wastes your strength." So again, as I pulled, the dark, magic whirlwind caught me, and she said, "You're doing beautifully; couldn't have done it better if you'd had a dozen babies!"

. . . After about two more thrilling pushes and a breath of oxygen, I heard the doctor say, "Hang on to this one and push the baby out." With the most spiraling, fascinating thrill of all, I felt the baby slither out. I wanted to shout with joy. Doctor held baby in her arms, baby cried, and I saw a perfect child attached to the cord. Doctor said reverently, "You have a little girl." . . . I wanted to stop and rest and drink in the thrill of having the baby. It was about five minutes before I wanted to push again. And then the last, slightly weaker, slightly less thrilling, but wonderful push, and out the placenta slipped.

. . . Bill walked with me to the elevator and I felt so good that I said, "It's silly to wheel me; I can walk. Bill, I feel as if I could do a day's washing right now." But after talking to him ten minutes in the maternity ward, I felt tired. He left—I started this letter, and then just rested.[20]

Does it seem a strange paradox that the birth of a child, which can cause such an agony of pain to a mother under certain conditions, can be a source of physical pleasure to her under other circumstances? Life is full of paradoxes. Love and hate are not so far apart as they seem, nor are tears and laughter. Sex itself carries the potentials of great pleasure, or great tragedy, uplifting or degrading, depending on the circumstances.

Some people may be shocked at the thought that the birth of a child can bring its mother physical pleasure. But what is their concept of the character of God? Is He a tyrant, who denies us pleasure, as some of our forefathers believed? Is He not rather a loving God, who delights in bringing pleasures to His children?

CONCLUSION

Adequate prenatal education is essential for a successful childbirth experience. Because of this, some members of the medical profession are now calling natural childbirth "psychophysical" or "psychosomatic" obstetrics. By this they mean that attention must be given to the "mind," *psychē*, as well as to the "body," *sōma*, of a pregnant woman. This is all right as far as it goes, but it leaves out the most essential component of a natural childbirth experience, which is *pneuma*, "spirit."

What the birth of this particular child means to me, the mother, is not just a matter of the mind, nor of the body, but is essentially a matter of the spirit. It is the spiritual significance of a birth that gives it dignity and beauty, for creativity is a spiritual function. Dr. Paul Tournier, in *The Meaning of Persons*, makes this distinction clear:

> The body and the mind are only the means of expression of the spirit, which co-ordinates and directs them both at once. The body and the mind which we study appear simply as mechanisms. . . . the instruments by means of which the spiritual reality which is the person expresses itself.
>
> . . . Dom Weisberger . . . expresses it thus: "To defend the person it is not enough to confine oneself to the specific nature of man as a composite mind-body, a reasoning animal. To defend the person is to defend man as being somebody . . . unique, incommunicable, irreplaceable, willed and loved by God. . . ."[21]

Two of us stand looking at a sunset. Our bodies are in the same place. Our mental perception is of the same scenery. But the *impression* that this sunset gives to each of us is individual, unique, a thing of the spirit. Though we have had the same mind-body experience, the spiritual significance will be different for each of us. If we each paint a picture of the sunset, these pictures will be different. They will reflect the spiritual perception and creativity of our own, unique personalities.

So it is with natural childbirth. Its principles have a universal application, for all women desire fulfillment in their childbearing experiences. But what this particular childbirth experience *means* to me is not just a matter of mind-body. It is a unique, personal, spiritual experience of creativity. Each woman is unique. Each child in a family is unique, different from his brothers and sisters. Giving birth to this particular child has a unique spiritual meaning to his mother, whether he is her first child or her tenth. It is this spiritual aspect which makes natural childbirth so rewarding.

> "She talks," I heard some say today,
> "As though none else had ever had a baby!"
> How right they are!
> No one else has ever borne this child, my husband's child.
> It is our own unique gift to the universe,
> The living symbol of our faith in the dignity of life,
> In the destiny of man,
> And in the reality of an eternal, living God.
> And God, Who made me for this hour,
> Will not desert me now!

Young women are most grateful for being taught how to give birth in a way in which it is to them a beautiful, personal, miracle. One young woman wrote, after the natural birth of her first child:

> Mrs. Wessel, I want you to know how grateful I am to you for all your helpful advice. . . . It has been such a blessing to me that I want to share my experience with others, too. So I have definitely made up my mind to try to help any expectant mother in our future pastorates to see that it can be a wonderful and blessed

experience. The natural way which the Lord intended it to be. I shall always be indebted to you and deeply appreciate it—more than you will ever know.

Another young woman, Shirley Martinez, wrote a thank-you to The American Institute of Family Relations for their prenatal classes. Her letter was first published in *Preparation for Parenthood News,* edited by Mary Jane Hungerford. When I wrote Mrs. Martinez for permission to quote her letter, she replied: "I'm so thrilled with natural childbirth that I'm willing to share my experience with others. It's an experience meant to be shared. Thank you for writing a book on the subject, and thank you for asking me to be a part of it." Mrs. Martinez' baby was a girl, her first child, and weighed 7 pounds, 8½ ounces:

> I am an RN and first saw "Natural Childbirth" as a student nurse ten years ago. After observing deliveries of all types, I had a chance to observe "Natural Childbirth," so asked to stay overtime and watch this mother's delivery. I was completely "sold." Could it be possible that labor, which to me before was accompanied by moaning, groaning and screaming, could be an experience that was capable of such powerful, exultant yet humble emotions? This patient was fully alert, was calm and confident throughout the whole first stage.
>
> I shall never forget the look on the woman's face as her baby was held up, still attached to the cord, to the mother who lost her first baby because of medication that made the baby so sluggish it died. The mother had a look of profound joy and her eyes filled with shining tears and her face looked as if a miracle had just happened to her. I remember as I stood there, that I had tears in my eyes too as did the other nurses, and I decided then and there, that if I ever got pregnant, I wanted to remember my baby's birth as this woman would, as an experience that was a beautiful miracle, not one of fright and pain from the contractions or a complete blank of the birth of the baby in second stage.
>
> My experience with "Natural Childbirth" was just as I hoped it would be, and I must admit tears flowed down my cheeks when I first saw my baby, I was so happy. There were 8 or 9 student nurses in the delivery room when I delivered, and like ten years

ago when I first saw "Natural Childbirth" and was "sold" on it, these students came to me later on in the maternity ward to say they were just thrilled with my delivery and the sight of joy on my face. They went to class after my delivery and told the rest of the class about it. They also said every student in the delivery room who watched the delivery wants to try it when they get pregnant, so as a nurse and as a mother, I want to say "Thank you" to the Institute for making my dream a reality.[22]

Should we not all stand humbled in awe at such evidence of God's love in our world, which has made such happiness possible? We can say with the Psalmist:

> Oh that men would praise the Lord for his goodness,
> And for his wonderful works to the children of men!
> For he satisfieth the longing soul,
> And filleth the hungry soul with goodness. . . .
> He turneth the wilderness into a standing water,
> And dry ground into watersprings. . . .
> He setteth the poor on high from affliction,
> And maketh him families like a flock.
> The righteous shall see it, and rejoice:
> And all iniquity shall stop her mouth.
> Whoso is wise, and will observe these things,
> Even they shall understand the loving kindness of the Lord.
> —Ps. 107:8, 9, 35, 41–43

Notes

1. Grantly Dick-Read, M.D., *Childbirth Without Fear*, 4th rev. ed. (New York: Harper & Row, 1972), p. 40.
2. Grantly Dick-Read, M.D., "The Birth of a Child," *Child-Family Digest*, June 1953. Reprinted by permission.
3. Charles D. Kimball, M.D., "An Evaluation of Family Centered Obstetrical Care," *The Western Journal of Surgery, Obstetrics and Gynecology*, Vol. 62, pp. 216-21, April 1954. Reprinted by permission.
4. A statement by M. Leonard Kimmel, M.D., in the panel discussion "Group Approaches to Childbirth Education," printed in the *ICEA 1962 Conference Report*, p. 83. Reprinted by permission.
5. "Letter from 'Natural Childbirth' Mother to Instructor," *Child-*

Family Digest, February 1952, pp. 49-51. Reprinted by permission.
6. Paul Tournier, M.D., *The Meaning of Persons* (New York: Harper, 1957), pp. 106, 107.
7. *A Correlation Chart for Expectant Parents and Their Attendants* (International Childbirth Foundation, 1960), p. 4.
8. Majorie Karmel, *Thank You, Dr. Lamaze* (Philadelphia and New York: Lippincott, 1959), p. 161.
9. Virginia Lawrence Larsen, M.D., "Comments" on the article "An Evaluation of Childbirth Training in Seattle," *Child-Family Digest,* May 1955, p. 79.
10. "I Want a Thousand Babies," *Child-Family Digest,* January 1952, pp. 94-99. Reprinted by permission.
11. Mrs. Grantly Dick-Read and Prunella Briance, *What Every Woman Should Know About Childbirth* (Grantly Dick-Read Childbirth Training Centre, 1960), p. 5. Reprinted by permission.
12. Grantly Dick-Read, M.D., "The Discomforts of Childbirth," the substance of a lecture delivered before St. Mary's Hospital Medical Society in October 1948, printed in the *British Medical Journal,* April 16, 1949, Vol. 1, p. 651.
13. Dick-Read, *What Every Woman Should Know About Childbirth,* p. 6. Reprinted by permission.
14. Dick-Read, *Childbirth Without Fear,* p. 230.
15. Michael Newton, M.D., and Niles Newton, Ph.D., "The Normal Course of Lactation," *Child and Family,* October 1962, pp. 6-12. Reprinted by permission.
16. Niles Newton, "The Sexual Implications of Breast Feeding," *Child-Family Digest,* November 1952, pp. 16-18. Reprinted by permission.
17. C. Lee Buxton, M.D., *A Study of Psychophysical Methods for Relief of Childbirth Pain* (Philadelphia: Saunders, 1962), p. 3. Reprinted by permission.
18. Marvin R. Weisbord, "Our Baby Wouldn't Wait to Be Born," *Reader's Digest,* June 1962, p. 138, condensed from "Our Baby Was Born at 30 M.P.H.," *Parents' Magazine,* March 1962.
19. N. Kalichman, M.D., "On Some Psychological Aspects of the Management of Labor," *The Psychiatric Quarterly,* Vol. 25, No. 4, 1951, pp. 655-71. Reprinted by permission.
20. "I Want a Thousand Babies," p. 97. Reprinted by permission.
21. Tournier, *The Meaning of Persons,* p. 169.
22. First printed in *Preparation for Parenthood News,* Mary Jane Hungerford, Ph.D., editor, by The American Institute of Family Relations, Los Angeles, Calif. Reprinted by permission.

Chapter 22

Breast-Feeding

MESSAGE TO PARENTS

I am your baby. I have just come from inner space where I was warm and held in a close, tight nest. I heard the rhythm of your heartbeat and felt the patting sensation that your breathing gave me. I was continuously tube fed; therefore, I was never in pain from hunger. I would occasionally drink the warm amniotic fluid that surrounded me. Maybe you noticed it when I had the hiccups. The thumbsucking that relatives object to—why, I have done that for months! I heard your voice and even Dad's when he came close to talk to me. I did not sleep all the time. You may have been aware of that fact when I had my exercise sessions—especially when you were lying on your back which meant I would be on your spine (squiggling or early creeping).

Please re-create for me the familiar surroundings of inner space. Allow me time to make the transition to outer space and to fulfill your expectations of what a baby is.

Feed me—I have never been hungry, or full.

Pat and stroke me. I'm used to this "touching."

Talk to me. Let me continue to hear your voice.

Hold me close. I was swaddled in the uterus and heard your heartbeat.

Look into my eyes. Let me study you and become acquainted with you.[1]

Breast-feeding is a baby's reassurance of security, feeling again the rhythm of the mother's breathing and heartbeat. This experience at her breast could be called "psychological birth," or the birth of love and acceptance, mother and baby giving and receiving warmth and love from each other as the baby's hunger is satisfied.

The physical benefits to the baby are immeasurable. Scientists are continually discovering new intrinsic values of breast milk. The milk not only contains immunoglobulin antibodies, which act against viruses and bacteria, but it is also easily digested and has the proper amount of lactose, protein, calcium, and other minerals. It has the proper biochemical balance for the human infant, an important factor to ecologically minded professionals and child-bearing couples.

Breast-feeding has been on the increase during the past few years, as knowledgeable young parents have increasingly rejected artificial feeding by bottle for their babies. These young people have been looking at life honestly and making choices objectively, refusing to follow blindly professional or traditional advice. They have cried out for peace rather than war, are rediscovering the positive values of nature, and are demanding clean air and water, natural foods, less wastefulness, more love for humanity. As the incidence of breast-feeding has increased there have been unexpected dividends for parents as well as for baby.

When the mother feeds her baby at her breasts, she experiences both psychological and physical benefits, for the two are closely interwoven. Dr. Deborah Tanzer in *Why Natural Childbirth?* writes:

> There are exceptionally close ties between reproductive and psychological functioning. We take for granted the influences of moods and feelings on courtship behavior and on sexual activity, as well as vice versa. . . . The interactions of body and mind in the woman's reproductive cycle are not at all surprising for there are events that start them, specific places in the body where they begin, pathways they follow and places where they end.
>
> The most obvious major pathway is the body's nervous system. . . . The involuntary nervous system . . . is intimately concerned with psychological activity, including emotions. It also provides the main direct nerve supply to the organs of the female reproductive system, especially the uterus. . . .

One neurohormone, oxytocin, is involved in mating behavior, birth and lactation or nursing. In orgasm, for example, oxytocin is thought to be related to contractions of the uterus. In labor and delivery, it helps stimulate uterine contractions. In breast feeding, it brings about "letdown"—release of the mother's milk. Particular smells, sights and sounds can send oxytocin out along internal pathways to stimulate specific responses. . . .[2]

When the baby touches the breast, or cries in anticipation of the breast, *oxytocin* is released from the mother's pituitary gland, which stimulates the uterus to contract pleasurably (as in female orgasm). This in turn stimulates the anterior lobe of the pituitary gland to release *prolactin*, a woman's built-in "tranquilizer." Many women have admitted a "baby-blues" period during the early weeks, when all the changes of daily life seem just too much. But there are honest, aware-of-themselves women who say, "Yes, a cloud of gloom did descend. But I just nursed my baby, and it went away!"

The disappearance of this depressed feeling was not just the result of cuddling the baby close and enjoying him but was also due to the release of *prolactin* into the bloodstream. Thus the best cure for a "nervous" mother is nature's built-in tranquilizer, released automatically into her system as her baby suckles at the breast.

The father has an extremely important supporting role in the breast-feeding family by his approving attitude, his reassurance that breast-feeding is best feeding, and his help with the chores. He will also be rewarded. He will share the joy that comes to his wife as she gains confidence in her role as an adequate mother. He will see her womanly beauty unfold as she nurses their baby and will also discover that nature is maturing her capacity as a sexual partner. And, of course, nature's tranquilizer, *prolactin*, released in her body as she breast-feeds, will make her a calmer mother and more pleasant to live with as a companion.

A man whose baby is breast-fed can hold the baby and help care for him as much as he has time for, without the infant ever confusing him with the mother! He need not keep his distance from the baby to prove his manliness.

PREPARATION FOR BREAST-FEEDING

Preparation for breast-feeding starts before the birth of the baby, both psychologically and physically. The person who has a mother who breast-fed, and who feels comfortable and natural about it, may have no psychological barrier to overcome. But the mother-to-be without this positive background will need to reassess her attitudes. Negative statements may come from well-meaning friends and relatives who have had poor experiences in breast-feeding or who are actually offended by the thought and cannot resist letting the expectant mother know how they feel.

The encouragement and support of the husband will offset the negativism of many of these people. It also helps to remember that their reactions only mirror their own dissatisfactions with themselves as women. In *Modern Motherhood*, Dr. Liley suggests:

> Breastfeeding is actually such an intimate part of our human life cycle that our reaction to the question reflects our approach to life. The proportion of women who breastfeed their babies is not so much a measure of our economics or sophistication as it is of our confidence and joy in motherhood.[3]

Physical preparation for breast-feeding begins six to eight weeks before the due date, and should be carried out even if the mother has previously nursed a baby. These simple exercises can be done during the daily showers or bath.

1. Breast Massage

> First use heat on the breasts to stimulate circulation and help you to relax. Direct the shower onto the breasts, or if in the bathtub, turn around and put your breasts into the water. If this position is awkward, place warm, wet washcloths on your breasts for ten minutes. Massage gently, as if a caress, around your breasts with the flat of your hands.
>
> Stimulation of the breasts in this manner causes the colostrum to be ejected. This is known as the "let-down" reflex. Express

the colostrum by grasping the breast between thumb and fingers behind the areolar (brown) area and squeeze gently but firmly. Work clockwise around the breast.

The purpose of this exercise is to set up free drainage of milk and prepare you for handling your breasts as you learn to nurse your baby. You will be less awkward and have more confidence.

2. Nipple-toughening Exercise

(a) Rub briskly with a bath towel as you dry yourself.

(b) Stretch areolar area outward with your thumbs moving in opposing directions. This will also stimulate the nipples to become erect, which will make the nipple-rolling exercise easier to carry out. This is also a good way to make a more pronounced nipple for your baby, when you do put baby to breast.

3. Nipple Roll

When the nipple is erect, support the breast with one hand, grasp the nipple of the breast that is being supported between your thumb and forefinger of the other hand, and roll the nipple back and forth.

Start with a count of 5 and gradually move up to a count of 20 on successive days. The purpose of this exercise is to toughen the nipples to prevent tenderness when you put baby to breast, and it also improves the erectibility of the nipples.

Questions pertaining to the breasts during pregnancy.

Q. What should I do about colostrum leaking when not doing this exercise?

A. If necessary to protect your clothing, wear commercial nursing pads or use white cleansing tissue, or men's white handkerchiefs. The amount of protection needed depends upon the amount of leaking.

Q. If I do not leak colostrum, does that mean that I will not have breast milk?

A. No. Women vary in the amount of leaking just as they vary after the birth in the amount of milk and the extent of leaking.

Q. How do I keep my nipples clean?

A. Occasionally the colostrum dries on the nipples and forms a slight crust. Soften this with a cream or a lanolin preparation and soak off gently as you bathe. Use a small amount of the cream after cleansing to prevent further "crusting" on the nipple, or to prevent the nipple from sticking to the breast pad.

MECHANICS OF BREAST-FEEDING

When the baby is put to breast for the first time, appreciate the fact that this is a new experience *for the baby*. It is possible that the new baby will go to breast and nurse vigorously, even immediately after birth. It is also possible that the baby will make very little response, and the mother may feel disappointed. So remember that the baby has just come from intrauterine life.

But the baby will learn amazingly fast, and it is for this reason that it is important for the new mother to use the proper methods in order to have the best experience for both. All mammals are *imprinted* orally soon after birth. Thus a baby fed only with a bottle the first few days may reject the mother's nipple when introduced to it later, for he has been imprinted with the feel of the rubber nipple. For the same reason a baby should be introduced to a bottle at least once during his first week, so that he will not reject it in an emergency, such as an unexpected illness or operation of the mother. Remember, imprinting occurs *early*.

A baby quickly develops his own oral habits, which are also imprinted, so it is important that these habits be set in the right direction from the very start. Remember, a mother may have breast-fed other babies BUT NOT THIS NEW BABY. Each baby is his own unique self with his very own oral mannerisms. Some habits, such as tongue sucking or thumb sucking, are already well established. Improper mechanics in breast-feeding at the outset can begin a self-defeating spiral of discouragement. The following suggestions will help establish a good breast-feeding experience for both mother and baby.

1. *Burp the baby before feeding.*
A baby that spits up after feeding may simply be bringing up milk on top of an air bubble that was not expelled before he began feeding.

2. *Uncover the baby's hands.*

It is important for the baby to have skin-to-skin contact with the mother by at least having his or her hands free to touch her breasts. It is even better if baby has on only a diaper and can lie against his mother's naked breast, while she strokes his whole body with her hands. This tactile stimulation of the baby's skin is most important for his best development.[4] A light blanket can be placed over both baby and mother to keep them from becoming chilled.

3. *Find a comfortable position.*

The most comfortable position for breast-feeding may be lying-down, sitting up in bed with a pillow to support the arm, or sitting in an armchair with the baby supported on a pillow.

The "football hold" for the baby while the mother is in a sitting position is amazingly comfortable. If you are right-handed, first hold the baby under your *right* arm as if he were a football, and put him onto your *right* breast. When it is time for him to feed on the *left* breast, hold him under your *left* arm while he nurses.

Many right-handed women tend to have a sore right nipple, because they attempt to put the baby onto the right breast while holding him with their less familiar left hand, across the front of their body. Consequently, the baby often does not get a proper grasp on the whole nipple and soreness results. (Conversely, left-handed women tend to develop a sore left nipple for the same reason, unless they adopt the "football hold.")

A *Caesarian-section mother* is also a surgical patient. She will need considerable assistance in positioning her baby comfortably, as well as some medication for pain to make her as relaxed as possible while breast-feeding during the first few days after the surgical delivery. The football hold is very comfortable for the Caesarean-section mother, when she can have her back rest straight up and the baby under her arm propped up on a pillow. The baby in this position puts no pressure on her abdomen.

A woman with *small breasts* will have an easier time breast-feeding if she sits up. Lying down flattens the breast and makes it more difficult for the baby to get a good hold on the nipple.

A woman who has *large breasts* will find the football hold very effective if she breast-feeds sitting up. (If she holds the baby in front of her in the conventional position, he will be "overpowered" with breasts and may become frustrated and not take the nipple.) Women with large breasts can also nurse their babies very well while lying on one side or the other, with the baby lying on the bed beside the breast.

4. *Vary the position used.*

A baby can become so accustomed to breast-feeding while lying down that he may refuse to nurse in any other position. Or a baby may develop a preference for one side over the other. This may be because of the way a mother moves her baby more smoothly and securely to one side compared with the other, or it may be that the nipple is more prominent and easier for him to grasp on the favored side. Unless the mother uses the football hold, a pattern is often seen of a right-handed mother observing that her baby prefers the left side, or vice versa for the left-handed mother.

5. *Alternate breasts each feeding.*

Start feeding on the breast you stopped on at the previous feeding. There is more stimulation on the first side and the nipple toughens more quickly, because a newborn sucks most vigorously on the first side on which he feeds. If each feeding begins on the same side, the baby will soon favor it over the other and perhaps refuse the other.

But if the breast on which feeding begins is alternated each time, each will receive the same amount of stimulation, and the baby is less likely to favor one side. An easy way to remember to alternate sides is to use a safety pin on the bra strap as a reminder. Start on the side with which you stopped at the last feeding.

6. *Take advantage of the "rooting reflex."*

This stimulus-response system is established before birth and aids the baby in finding the nipple and grasping it correctly. Stroke the baby's mouth with your nipple. The "rooting reflex" will cause the baby to turn *toward the side stroked*, open his mouth and put his tongue down.

Wait until there is a wide open-mouthed response, as with a baby bird, and check carefully to be sure the tongue is *down* and not up on the roof of the baby's mouth.

Remember that if you try to push baby's cheek toward the nipple with your finger, the rooting reflex will make him turn *toward your finger* instead, and away from the breast. He instinctively turns his face *toward* the touch he feels.

By taking advantage of the rooting reflex, waiting until the baby's mouth is wide open and his tongue down, it is possible for him to take the whole nipple area into his mouth rather than just taking the tip and working his way onto the nipple. When a baby is allowed to nuzzle at the nipple and work his way onto it, he will often end up just sucking on the tip, and not on the areolar area around it that would stimulate the milk. This is the "drip" method of eating and is a frequent cause for sore nipples. It will take longer to satisfy the baby, and he may just roll his tongue around the tip of a nipple and suck on it as a pacifier without getting much milk. He will gain slowly, and before long the milk supply will diminish because of lack of proper stimulation.

Keep in mind that a baby is continuously nourished in the uterus by means of the blood vessels in the umbilical cord, so that he has never been hungry or full before. The transition to being fed after birth is in the mother's control. She should realize that the baby has been swallowing amniotic fluid, so that swallowing fluid is not new to him, *but* the manner in which it is now to be done is new.

A baby who has been sucking his thumb or tongue in the uterus may attempt to continue this type of tongue action habit the first times at the breast. A baby who has been tongue sucking before birth must be trained to suck with his tongue *down* UNDER the mother's nipple. One of the frequent causes of sore nipples is due to sucking by a baby whose tongue is above the nipple, damaging the nipple and providing no milk for him. Although his gums are around the nipple, he is still sucking only his own tongue. In the tongue-sucking position, the baby dimples its cheeks and is on the breast with the tongue thrusting above the nipple.

Tongue sucking while on the breast is a totally negative experience. The mother quickly has a very sore nipple. The baby is not learning how to eat in the world outside the uterus, and the mother will become engorged. The baby also loses being nourished with the very valuable colostrum that nature has planned for the first zero to three days of life.

7. *The proper pump-swallow action.*

When the baby is nursing well with the nipple fully grasped in his mouth, one can feel and hear the productive pumping action. The jaw is thrust upward, milk is expressed, and the baby swallows. The action of his jaws around the areolar area above the nipple not only draws the milk more adequately but also stimulates the mother's milk supply.

8. *The "let-down" reflex.*

If the mother is relaxed, she will "let down" the milk. The baby cannot suck out the milk until the mother "lets" it come down. If she is inhibited or upset or has difficulty relaxing, then she should use the abdominal (sleep) breathing she used to relax during pregnancy and labor. As she lets go of muscle tension and breathes more deeply and quietly, the milk will be able to come down.

9. *Time at the breast.*

Many mothers think that a newborn is still hungry when she removes him from her breast after the allotted time, and he cries. A newborn enjoys being held close and he enjoys sucking. But he takes 90 per cent of the feeding in the first seven minutes of breast feeding, so that it is not necessary for him to remain at the breast.[5] If his sucking needs are not satisfied, he can still be held close, and given a pacifier.

It is extremely important to limit the time at the breast at first, to avoid the nipples becoming sore. It is much better to feed a newborn for short periods of time, eight to ten times in twenty-four hours, than to feed him a few times for long periods. Frequent stimulation increases milk production and an easy flow, preventing problems of engorgement. And short periods of breast feeding allow tender nipples opportunity to adjust.

A suggested guide is to increase gradually the amount of time from two to three minutes each time at the breast the first day, up to ten minutes per session by the time the baby is seven days old.

10. *Breaking suction.*

A baby literally creates suction as he nurses. The selling point for plastic disposable bottles is based on this fact, for as the baby withdraws milk from the bottle, it collapses. A vacuum is being created. A similar condition is present in breast feeding.

The most effective way to break this suction is by inserting the little finger between the *gums* of the baby, where the vacuum is being created. It is NOT enough to slip a finger into the corner of his mouth. A vigorously nursing baby can easily create sore nipples if a mother pulls him off the breast incorrectly. Ease your baby off the breast as you break the suction of his gums.

11. *Caring for the nipples after feeding.*

After feeding the newborn, leave the nipples exposed to the air for at least fifteen minutes. If they are tender, this can be continued for an indefinite period of time. A 25-watt bulb at eight inches distance will hasten healing on a tender nipple, providing a source of warmth along with the air drying. (At home, hair dryers can be used rather than a light bulb, or sunlight.)

Redheads, blondes or women who burn easily are more likely to have tender nipples when first breast-feeding. Mild nipple cream such as Nivea or Massé may be used in these cases after the air and/or light drying of the nipples, but should be used *sparingly*. It is not meant to coat the nipple. A small amount is to be worked into the tissue. These are water-soluble creams that will not hinder the natural secretions being excreted from the nipple.

12. *Meditate on making milk.*

As the new mother gains confidence in her new role of breast-feeding, she will become more relaxed. This in turn will assure her of an optimum breast-feeding experience. Her great imperative from the time of birth is to relax and MEDITATE ON MAKING MILK.

There is no one from a dairy-farming background who does not appreciate the fact that a milking cow will not "give" milk if there is a tension-producing factor, such as turbulent weather, a stranger trying to milk the cow, or even a stranger in the barn. At the time of the San Francisco earthquake in 1906 it was reported that the cows in the area did not give milk for three days.

If animals feel tension, how much more so do human beings, who have so many other causes for stress. The adrenalin triggered by the autonomic nervous system in response to stress actually inhibits the release of the chemical oxytocin. Since it is oxytocin that causes the tissue around the milk glands to contract, there is no "let-down" reflex or milk ejection if the oxytocin is inhibited. And if there is no "let-down," there is no milk when baby sucks.

When no inhibiting factor is present, within a few days to a week after birth the let-down reflex will be quickly stimulated by the baby at the breast. It may be that as baby nurses on one breast, let-down of milk occurs from the other breast also and it begins to leak milk. Or the let-down may occur when the mother hears her baby cry, or hears ANY baby cry. Even looking at the baby or thinking about him may cause the milk to begin flowing.

The let-down reflex can also be stimulated by the husband caressing his wife's breast. What happens in this amazing process is that when the nipple is stimulated either by the baby or by the husband's touch, the posterior lobe of the pituitary gland is stimulated to release the oxytocin. When breast-feeding women resume intercourse, this same mechanism may be stimulated. One pro-breast-feeding doctor has remarked that the "let-down" reflex of milk leaking during mating is truly an indication of sexual response to one's husband!

But if a woman is "uptight," adrenalin inhibits the stimulating signal of baby or husband from reaching the brain, the oxytocin is not released and there is no let-down of milk. With no letting-down, no prolactin is released—the important substance that creates the tranquil feeling occurring as a mother breast-feeds or following orgasm.

If the mother is tense, unable to let down her milk, she should consciously relax all her muscles and use abdominal "sleep" breathing. As the baby takes the nipple, it may help for the husband to gently caress her breasts, since this sexual stimulation may help release the necessary oxytocin.

When not breast-feeding, it helps one to relax by using heat, perhaps in the bathtub, turning around and placing the breasts into the water, or placing warm washcloths on them. Hot-water bottles or an electric heating pad may help at other times, for heat stimulates the circulation as well as aiding relaxation. Sometimes a cup of tea will help. Anything that puts the mother into a relaxed mood before breast-feeding will aid the let-down reflex so that the baby is amply rewarded for his sucking efforts.

PROBLEMS

1. *Sore nipples.*

Any time there is a tender or bleeding nipple there is a mechanical failure in the procedure used. Try to discover what is causing the problem.

Check the position of the baby's tongue. Make sure he is well onto the areola around the nipple and that his tongue is down under the nipple and not above it.

Breast-feed more often and for shorter periods of time until the nipples are toughened. If baby needs additional milk, express some directly into his mouth.

Remember to break the suction of the baby's gums before taking him off the breast. Air-dry the nipples for longer periods of time to hasten the toughening process. Apply cream after the air drying. For women with light-colored nipples it is well to toughen them with a nipple cream (such as Massé or Nivea) during the six to eight weeks before the birth, too.

If a nipple is very sore, a rubber breast shield such as "Breast-Eze" can be used over the nipple to protect it as baby feeds. This type of nipple cover is also used for inverted nipples, those that are broad, flat and poorly defined, or for nipples too large for a baby with a very small mouth. The nipple shield should be used no longer than necessary, however, because of the problem of imprinting the baby to it, so that he rejects the mother's natural nipple.

If the skin is broken and there is bleeding, it is better to take the baby off the breast for twenty-four hours. The milk can be hand-expressed and given to him in a bottle. Spend ample time air-drying the nipples with a light bulb or other mild source of heat (hairdryer, sunlight) to hasten healing.

2. *Engorgement.*

This is the term used to describe the massive congestion in the breasts that may occur during the first week to ten days. The engorgement occurs for several reasons:

  1. The veins in the breasts have an increased supply of blood due to hormonal changes, and circulation may become sluggish. This creates pressure so that fluid from the blood vessels seeps into surrounding tissues.
  2. The lymph ducts bring additional fluid to the breasts.
  3. The milk that is collecting in the breasts is not totally or evenly withdrawn by the sleepy newborn, and the collecting pools of milk in the breast become filled.

A woman in this condition is in considerable pain. She is frustrated because it is now difficult to put the baby to breast, for it is so full the nipple no longer extends. The baby is also upset, for he is unable to grasp the nipple and areola.

This does not need to happen! *Do not allow your breasts to become too hard.* Apply heat to the breasts as previously described, breast-feed more frequently to draw off the excess milk, and follow the techniques for relaxing to allow let-down of the milk. (The doctor may prescribe Syntocinon nasal spray for you—a synthetic oxytocic—to aid the let-down reflex.)

Massage the breasts, placing both hands flat on the breast well above it and press down, moving the hands down over the breasts. (Do not touch the areola or nipple but glide over them.) Next, place hands underneath the breast with thumbs above and again press gently, gliding hands toward the nipple area. Apply pressure in this way evenly all around the breast. Repeat on the other breast. Remember to massage *gently*, as a caress. It may help to have the husband massage the breasts. His touch will help stimulate the let-down reflex.

After massaging, express the colostrum or milk by pressing with thumbs and forefingers above and below the areola (not *on* it), in a gentle scissors or squeezing motion. Then move the thumb and forefinger a quarter turn and repeat. At the same time, use the other hand to press down gently but firmly on the breast above the areola, all the way around, especially on any portion that feels lumpy, like little "moth balls" in the breast, for the glands are deep. There are fifteen to twenty milk glands around the breast, which fill with milk—like little balloons. Each of these glands leads to a separate duct. It is important to empty these little "balloons" and to keep the ducts open so that the milk will flow freely.

Each time after breast-feeding the baby, express milk from any area of the breast that feels hard or is not comfortable. If the newborn does not take from the second breast at a feeding, express enough from this breast to keep it soft. Many have asked, "If I keep expressing, won't it make more milk?" The answer is NO. The mother is overproducing for this particular baby and needs to express enough to keep good drainage and remain comfortable.

If engorgement occurs, *do not use ice packs* on the breasts. Heat is needed, to increase circulation. Do not use a breast pump for early engorgement. It is both ineffective and painful. (Later on, a breast pump will be all right). Also be careful not to wear a brassière that is too tight.

3. *Overproduction of milk.*

Since breast milk is on a supply-demand basis, milk is made as the breasts are stimulated, but it takes a little while for the baby's needs and mother's supply to be in balance. Skipping a feeding will cut down on stimulation, but if you do offer the baby a bottle, be sure to express enough milk to keep the breasts soft. It is better to extend the time between breast feedings rather than to give the baby a bottle.

It may be that the baby needs more sucking but not more food. If he seems to have an insatiable need for sucking, use a correctly shaped pacifier (like the NUK Sauger Exerciser) to satisfy his need, but do not let him use your breasts as pacifiers, sucking endlessly.

When overproducing, it may be that when let-down occurs a sudden ejection of milk will come so fast that the baby cannot swallow fast enough, and will cough or choke. Some babies will pull back off the breast. Others will stay on, but will gulp-eat because of the forceful flow of milk, gulping air along with the milk.

A baby who gulp-feeds may spit up the whole feeding. If he doesn't, he may be "gassy" or fussy after eating, not digest the feeding properly, and have greenish stools with an unpleasant odor. When it is apparent that the baby is choking, pulling back, coughing, or noisily gulp-eating, break the suction and remove him from the breast. Burp him and then express enough milk to slow down the flow before putting him back to breast.

4. *Leaking breasts.*

This profound "letting-down" may not continue the entire time that you breast-feed. It varies with different women. Some women leak milk only at first, and after the supply is stabilized leaking does not occur. Use breast pads according to your need, flannel squares, folded men's handkerchiefs, or cut-up sanitary napkins. The pads should be of material that will not seal off the air.

5. *Undersupply of milk.*

The milk is produced in response to stimulation. The more frequently a baby nurses, the more stimulation there will be. If you do not seem to have enough milk, take a look first at your own needs. Are you getting enough *rest*? Are you "uptight" about something? Be sure you are drinking ten to twelve glasses of fluid a day, including some milk, and eat a balanced diet of vegetables, fruit, dairy products, fish, nuts, meat and grains (bread, cereal).

Make certain the baby is up onto the areola well and pumping productively, not just sucking on the nipple tip without stimulating the milk supply.

A boy baby is often circumcised on the day the mother's milk begins to replace the colostrum. The baby is tired following this experience and may not nurse well, and the mother may feel a bit low due to the hormonal changes in her body after the birth. At such a time the first-time, breast-feeding mother may become pessimistic about ever breast-feeding properly. She may panic, thinking, "I can't nurse my baby! There's no milk. I'm starving my baby!" Or she may worry if she has ample milk, and he won't breast-feed.

If this occurs, give yourself the day to *relax* and enjoy your baby, learning to become a mother. Your internal chemistry *will* adjust to his needs if you are patient and follow the suggestions given. A baby does not need a large amount of food immediately and is in no danger of starving. If the milk is in and baby won't breast-feed that day, hand-express the milk to keep the breasts soft.

At six weeks of age, and again at three months, a baby has a growth spurt and may suddenly demand more milk than is being produced. When this occurs, take a day off and MEDITATE ON MAKING MILK. Breast-feed him every two hours, rest, and soon your supply will increase enough to satisfy his new demands.

If you become ill or the baby is sick, this will temporarily cut down on the supply. If you must be separated, keep expressing the milk, and then nurse more frequently again when you are reunited. If hospitalization is required, mother and baby should be allowed to remain together if at all possible. It is a simple fact that *you need each other* to keep each other comfortable.

6. *Common questions.*

Q. My baby lost weight. Was it because my milk was not rich enough?

A. No. If you are tense or tired, the milk in the breasts is not letting-down to the baby, and he will lose weight. Rest more, and use the suggestions for increasing the milk supply. Remember that almost all new babies lose weight the first few days.

Q. I know my milk is not rich enough because it is so thin and bluish-looking.

A. The colostrum that is present the first three days of the baby's life is rich and creamy looking. When the milk comes in, it appears watery by comparison. But it has all the elements the baby needs from his mother.

Q. I had "the shot" to dry up my breasts. Now I want to breast-feed. Is it possible?

A. *Yes.* The shot does not inhibit milk production but is used as a medication to cut down the painful engorgement period. Put baby to breast frequently, and it will stimulate your supply adequately.

Q. Why did my baby keep spitting up and having gas? Was my milk too rich for him?

A. The milk flow may have been coming too fast so that he gulped air as he swallowed. Express a little milk before feeding so that he need not gulp-swallow.

Q. My breasts are too small for breast feeding.
A. Size has nothing to do with one's ability to breast-feed. Every woman has milk glands. The size of breast varies only in the amount of fatty tissue present, and has nothing to do with milk glands.

Q. The doctor said the baby was allergic to my milk. He had a rash, so the doctor put him on soybean milk.
A. Take a look at your diet and eliminate or take smaller amounts of those foods that cause a reaction in your baby, such as a rash, diarrhea, throwing up, green stools with a bad odor, or gasiness. (Foods that make you "gassy" will affect baby, too.) It is better to avoid sugars, chocolates, pickles, garlic, too rich or spicy foods, or an excess of any one food.

Q. After I got home with the baby, I lost my milk.
A. The heavy, full feeling in the breast disappears after the first week to ten days, and the breasts become softer. There is just as much milk, but the excess swelling of the surrounding tissues has gone down.

Q. My baby got constipated from being breast-fed and did not have a bowel movement for several days.
A. Babies differ considerably in their stools. After birth, the color of the stools changes from black to green to greenish-yellow to yellow. The consistency will vary from loose to "curdy" or pasty. Some babies will have a stool after every feeding. Others may even go for several days, and then, when it occurs, will have a massive stool of soft consistency.

TRANSITIONS

1. In the hospital a baby may fall asleep and be content after nursing from only one breast. Once you are at home, wake your baby to feed on the second breast, too—unless you do not mind feeding him every hour. Because a baby has never been hungry or full before, he nurses only to a comfortable feeling. A mother is soft and warm; he hears her heartbeat again and her rhythmic

breathing as he nurses, and falls asleep. If you put the baby down at this point, he may wake up and cry immediately.

Program your baby to this world by waking him up after feeding on the first side. Change the diapers before feeding him on the second breast, or give him a bath, or rub his feet, or loosen his clothing first. In general, make him less cozy and comfortable so that he will be alert enough to continue breast-feeding on the second breast. (Remember to burp him first.)

2. It is no great achievement to have the baby sleep through the night. As he matures, he will sleep longer periods of time. If he wakens during the night, perhaps the daddy will get up, change him and bring him to the mother to breast feed in bed. Return the baby to his own bed when he has finished nursing.

3. Do not try to be a hostess on your arrival home, but concentrate on being a mother, and give yourself time to adjust to your new role. If there are people who insist on visiting, your husband should "run interference" for you. *You* are your baby's best mother. Be kind to your new little son or daughter by being kind to yourself.

4. Breast feeding is not 100 per cent assurance that you will not ovulate. If you are TOTALLY breast-feeding, you may not ovulate; the prolactin is thought to inhibit ovulation, so that no egg is discharged from the ovary. Just because you are not menstruating does not mean you are not ovulating.

It is not wise to take birth control pills while breast-feeding, as it may affect your milk supply. Talk over with your husband and doctor what forms of family planning you may want to consider.

5. Solid foods (soft cereal, strained fruits and vegetables) are not necessary for the breast-feeding baby before he is three months old. Some authorities suggest that no solids are necessary before six months. When you do begin offering solids, breast-feed first on one side, offer the solids, then breast-feed on the second side. As baby's intake of solid foods increases, the milk supply will diminish.

6. Weaning need not occur before the baby is several months

old. He can be trained to drink from a cup long before weaning from the breast is necessary, taking juice or water by cup.

Some babies continue breast-feeding into the second or even into the third year once or twice a day. Children eventually wean themselves, if the weaning is not forced on them earlier. Let your child's needs be your guide. But be sure that weaning occurs gradually, since this makes the adjustment easier for both you and your child.

In some cultures children have been breastfed even longer than two or three years. There is nothing wrong with this, although it seems unusual to . In Bible times children were often breastfed well beyond th irst year of life. Isaiah asks, "Can a woman forget her sucking ild? . . ." (Isa. 49:15.)

The child Samuel was breastfed until he was old enough to wear special garments and run errands for Eli the priest, so that he would need to have been at least three years old before the weaning occurred.

> And when she weaned him, she took him up with her, and the child was young. . . . And they brought the child to Eli . . . Samuel ministered before the Lord, being a child, girded with a linen ephod. Moreover his mother made him a little coat, and brought it to him from year to year, when she came up with her husband to offer the yearly sacrifice. (I Sam. 1:22–2:19.)

Notes

1. Ilene S. Rice, *A Breastfeeding Guide* (St. Joseph's Hospital, St. Paul, Minn.), p. 1. Reprinted by permission.
2. Deborah Tanzer, Ph.D. and Jean L. Block, *Why Natural Childbirth?* (Garden City, N.Y.: Doubleday, 1972), pp. 60–62. Reprinted by permission.
3. M. M. I. Liley, M.D. and Beth Day, *Modern Motherhood* (New York: Random House, 1966), p. 19. Reprinted by permission.
4. Ashley Montagu, *Touching, The Human Significance of the Skin* (New York: Columbia University Press, 1971).
5. *The Womanly Art of Breastfeeding* (Franklin Park, Ill.; La Leche League, 1963).

Chapter 23

The New Family

There was a child went forth every day,
And the first object he look'd upon, that object he became,
And that object became part of him for the day
    or certain part of the day,
Or for many years or stretching cycles of years. . . .
His own parents, he that had father'd him and she that had
    conceiv'd him in her womb and birth'd him.
They gave this child more of themselves than that,
They gave him afterward every day, they became part of him.

The mother at home quietly placing the dishes on the
    supper-table,
The mother with mild words, clean her cap and gown, a wholesome
    odor falling off her person and clothes as she walks by,
The father, strong, self-sufficient, manly, mean, anger'd
    unjust,
The blow, the quick loud word, the tight bargain, the
    crafty lure,
The family usages, the language, the company, the furniture,
    the yearning and swelling heart,
Affection that will not be gainsay'd, . . .
                                            ——Walt Whitman

A family is not just a group of individuals living together, but an interacting unit, modifying and shaping each others' lives. The Bible says, "None of us lives to himself, and none of us dies to himself" (Rom. 14:7 RSV), and this is especially true in the family setting.

Families are under stress these days, with husband, wife and children struggling for their own identity, restless for "rights," "freedom," "equality," "independence." While these goals are admirable, they can be achieved only in *relation to* other human beings, for they are not the goals of an individual living in complete isolation.

Families ought not to exist to keep their members from these goals but to make their attainment possible for each member. Childbirth experiences are not the only factors in determining the extent of intimate harmony and peace within the family unit, with each member free to discover his or her own creative potential, for basic attitudes toward life precede the birth experience and are only reinforced by it in one direction or the other. It is thus likely that the couple with a healthy attitude toward childbearing and breast-feeding, who have prepared for and shared the joy of these experiences, will be a couple who have already made a good adjustment to each other as husband and wife. Their relationship will not have been only in coitus but in responding to each other in every aspect of daily living, in the very special companionship of marriage.

But when a child enters that home, his coming disrupts the male/female balance. It is no longer a "couple" but is now a "family," in which there are two females and one male, or two males and one female. A complex set of relationships has begun, which the new parents need to think through carefully, in relation to each other as well as in relation to the new baby.

For the fetus *in utero* there is no sexual differentiation in the early weeks. The basic tendency of the human fetus is to develop as a female. Unless the genes order the gonads to become testicles and produce the male hormone androgen, the embryo will not turn into a boy but will become a girl. Something has to be added in the process of development to create a male.[1]

Thus the new baby is not yet primarily male or female. He is primarily a *person*. But from the time of birth others may unconsciously respond to him or her in terms of his or her sexuality, disappointed that it's a boy, disappointed that it's a girl, happy that it's a boy, happy that it's a girl, placing more importance on the child's sex than on his or her essential personhood. Subtle pressures to conform to society's expectations of one sex or the other begin early. We see the tragic consequences in the high incidence of homosexuality prevalent and in the trend toward sex-change operations. Often these unhappy people have not been accepted as individuals but have been forced into an arbitrary cultural role that they were not born to fit. Their potential "personhood" has been violated.

This does not mean that there are not differences in the infant and small child, both of temperament and of interests, that may reflect his sex. But the child who is secure in the knowledge of being accepted as a person is better able to accept his or her own sexual identity with pride when that awareness begins to dawn.

And if the parents are to be able to accept their new baby as a person rather than as "just" a boy or girl, it would be wise for them to take another look at themselves as man and woman, both in relation to each other as well as to the baby, reaffirming the essential personhood of both husband and wife.

FIRST A PERSON

The Bible makes it clear that we are male or female only secondarily. We are persons first, human beings with equal capacity for spiritual and intellectual growth and the development of creative capabilities. Genesis 1:27 says:

> God said, "Let us make mankind (*adam*) in our image. . . . So God created man in his own image; male and female created he them.

If mankind (man and woman) is in God's image, what is that "image"? Jesus explains it for us when He says, "God is a *Spirit,* and those who worship him must worship in spirit and in truth" (John 4:24). Thus the first element of personhood is not flesh and blood but "spirit," a creative personality.

Religious leaders once tried to trap Jesus with a question about the role of men and women after death (Matt. 22:23-30), citing the hypothetical case of a woman who had been widowed seven times. To which man would she belong in heaven? Jesus' reply was that their question was foolish. "You don't know either the Scripture, or the power of God," He said, "for in the resurrection they neither marry nor are given in marriage, but are like the angels in heaven" (who are neither male nor female).

Paul says in Gal. 3:28: "There is neither Jew nor Greek, there is neither slave nor free, there is *neither male nor female*; for you are all one in Christ Jesus" (RSV).

Our creative personality, our real "self," our "spirit," is not bound by the limitations of sex. Only the body, which houses the spirit, comes in male or female form. The essential "personhood" of man and woman is the same.

The early Church leaders were careful to explain this. In Chapter 17, "Evidences From Anthropology," some of their statements were given. Here are a few more:

Clement of Rome (A.D. 30-100)

> Many women also, being strengthened by the grace of God, have performed numerous manly exploits.[2]

Clement of Alexandria (A.D. 153-217)

> Let us, then, embracing more and more this good obedience, give ourselves to the Lord . . . and understand that the virtue of man and woman is the same. For if the God of both is one, that master of both is also one; one church, one temperance, one modesty; their food is common, marriage an equal yoke; respiration, sight, hearing, knowledge, obedience, love all alike.

> And those whose life is common have common graces and a common salvation; common to them are love and training. "For in this world," he says, "they marry and are given in marriage." in which alone the female is distinguished from the male; "but in that world it is so no more."

> There the rewards of this social and holy life, which is based on conjugal union, are laid up, not for male and female, but for man, the sexual desire which divides humanity being removed. . . .[3]

Obviously, the equal worth of a man and woman does not mean "sameness," nor do their physical differences imply superiority or inferiority as persons. There are some personality differences that reflect sex, but these are not nearly as great as we have often been led to believe.

Female hormones not only make the body softer, rounder, but also tend to make women quieter, more receptive, more conscious of people than of things. Male hormones may make a man more restless, aggressive, explorative, more often goal-oriented than person-oriented.[4] However, although male/female hormones affect temperament to a certain degree, we must not forget that every normal person is a blend of male/female qualities. The differences are a matter of *degree* rather than absolute. In God we see the perfect blend of these traits, aggressiveness without hostility, tenderness without weakness.

The temperament of a man or a woman does not just reflect the dominant hormones in their body but is also affected by his or her intellect and interests, according to the unique make-up of the individual.

> Women are often referred to in one way or another as "chemical creatures" with resulting mood changes. With the consistent absence of any accompanying discussion of the same phenomenon in men, one could easily conclude that men are relatively immune from such characteristics. There is, however, no sociological, physiological or scriptural basis for this implication. To the contrary, the often ignored but richly documented fact is that men have a pronounced 30-day hormone level rhythm with mood cycles of four to six weeks in duration.[5]
>
> Overall it is necessary to realize that *both* men and women respond to stresses differently at various times of the month. Fortunately these changes can be modified and even minimized by meaningful and satisfying relationships and activities.[6]

As persons, men and women are endowed with a variety of intellectual and creative potentials. The differences in the creative potential of any individual is not related to his or her sexuality but to the gifts he has inherited from both parents, which may or may not have the opportunity to flourish, depending on the culture into which one is born and the family's position in that culture.

The importance of sexual roles is primarily in relationship to others, both within the family and to society at large within a given cultural setting.

Cultural Differences

In every culture there is a division of labor, but these divisions have not been consistent with sexual differences. In some cultures women have done all the manual labor while the men have been left free for hunting expeditions or for sudden defense against attack by neighboring tribes. In other cultures only the "poor" have worked at manual labor, while both men and women in the upper classes considered it disgraceful to use their hands at daily tasks. In such cultures, men and women servants worked in the kitchen and cared for the children, while both men and women servants toiled in the fields.

Because of such cultural variables, one cannot use Biblical statements as blanket proof of certain prevalent attitudes, such as "woman's place is in the home." Even a brief glance at the cultural settings in Bible times shows that this claim is not valid. People lived in extended families, with relatives next door or close by in the village, if not under the same roof, so that children were under the care of familiar persons all the time. In more prosperous homes both men and women performed many of the tasks, indoors and out. In poorer homes everyone worked, in the fields and in the market.

The "ideal wife" of Proverbs 31 is a beautiful example of a "working wife." She helped support the household with her income as a manufacturer, as a merchant who sold her wares in the public market, as a buyer of real estate, and as a farmer who "planted a vineyard with her own hands." Who took care of the children and housework while she was busy with all these business activities? Baby-sitters, of course. "She rose early in the morning to appoint tasks for her maidens."

Grandmothers, rather than the mother, often cared for the small children. When Ruth married Boaz, her baby was given to the grandmother Naomi to care for. "Naomi took the child and laid him in her bosom, and became his nurse" (Ruth 4:16). This was not unusual.

In poorer homes women worked outside along with the men.

Before marrying Boaz, Ruth harvested in the fields along with the regular farm workers, who were both men and women (Ruth 2:3-9).

Frequently, Paul's teaching in I Tim. 5:11-14 is quoted to prove that women are to be kept at home, but this could not be what Paul meant. In his time many women *had* to work out of sheer economic necessity. Priscilla[7] worked right along with Paul and Aquila manufacturing tents. Paul's teaching is that young women should not be allowed to be "*idle*, gadding about from house to house, and not only idlers but gossips and busybodies" (RSV).

If he could see how many wives live today, spending idle hours on the phone or at coffee parties or running to "sales," he would say that these idle young women would be better off finding useful employment.

Another fallacy is that women are more emotional than men and thus not suited to public life. However, emotions are a part of being human, not of being female. The way emotions are *expressed* is culturally determined rather than determined by sex. In current society it is considered unmanly for a man to cry or to show his feelings in public (though not unmanly for him to develop ulcers or headaches from repressed emotions). Only women are expected to let their feelings show.

> . . . cultural factors render boys and men more vulnerable to a whole spectrum of pressures . . . his assigned sex *role*—what people expect of him—puts him at a psychological disadvantage as well. . . .
>
> Women may be "more emotional," but more men are emotionally *disturbed*. (All over the world, more males than females have nervous breakdowns, more males than females commit suicide.) Biology again? A weaker nervous system? Perhaps. But it may be that women's very freedom to *be* emotional, to show and express their feelings, permits them to let off steam, while men are expected to sit on their emotions. No safety valve—hence, *bang!*[8]

Jesus did not hide his tears and was not afraid to show tenderness in public. In Bible times it was most often the *men* who made public displays of emotion, weeping loudly, kissing and embracing other men in public, indulging openly in sorrow (Gen. 33:4; II Sam. 18:35; 19:4; Luke 15:20; Acts 20:36,37).

Still another mistaken concept is that women are psychologically and spiritually more gullible than men. Yet it was to the male religious leaders of His day that Jesus gave His harshest pronouncements, with statements such as "You blind guides! hypocrites! deceived and deceivers!" (Matt. 23; John 9:41).

Women were among the disciples of Jesus throughout His earthly ministry (Matt. 27:55) and followed Him all the way to the cross even when the disciples had deserted Him (Luke 23:27,55,56). Women were first at the tomb and the first to see the risen Lord (Luke 24:10,11, John 20:11–18), but when they told this to the men, "these words seemed to them an idle tale, and they did not believe them."

Women were among the hundred and twenty at the first Pentecost. When Paul later had a vision of a man calling him to Macedonia, he obeyed. And what did he find? Only a bunch of women down by the riverside. The first European convert was one of these women, Lydia, a businesswoman.

Only when we understand the essential capacity for development of the unique personhood of husband, wife, child, without false cultural impositions, are we ready to look objectively at their relationship to each other within the family. There is a Biblical standard for these relationships that will not only make harmonious living together possible but when correctly carried out will in no way inhibit the unique flowering of the creative potential of any of the family members. On the contrary, it will enhance it.

The Biblical standard is found in Eph. 5:21; 6:4 (RSV):

> Be subject to one another out of reverence for Christ. Wives, be subject to your husbands, as to the Lord. For the husband is the head of the wife as Christ is the head of the church, his body, and is himself its Savior. As the church is subject to Christ, so let wives be subject in everything to their husbands.
>
> Husbands, love your wives, as Christ loved the church and gave himself up for her, . . . Even so husbands should love

their wives as their own bodies. He who loves his wife loves himself. For no man ever hates his own flesh, but nourishes and cherishes it, as Christ does the church, because we are members of his body. . . .

Children, obey your parents in the Lord, for this is right. "Honor your father and mother" (this is the first commandment with a promise), "that it may be well with you and that you may live long on the earth."

Fathers, do not provoke your children to anger, but bring them up in the discipline and instruction of the Lord.

LOVING HUSBANDS

God is not only a Creative Spirit but a threefold Being, who said (Gen. 1:27), "Let *us* make mankind in *our* image. . . ." The Father, Son and Holy Spirit, co-equal, co-existant, co-eternal, God in Three Persons, are in a *relationship* with one another. The Son, though equal with the Father, willingly places Himself under the will of the Father (Phil. 2:3–11). The Holy Spirit, though equal with the Father and the Son, willingly places Himself at the disposal of the Son (John 1:33; 16:7).

In a human family, though each member is of equal worth, there is a definite hierarchy of responsibility to be willingly carried out for the good of all. But the entire family is under the authority of God, with whom they are *not* equal.

The husband is under the authority of Christ, who shows him by His own example how a husband is to "lead" his wife. Only those are fit to lead who have first learned to obey their own leader. The Scripture says that the husband is the "head of the wife" (I Cor. 11:3) and the "ruler of his household" (I Tim. 3:4), but there is no command in Scripture for him to "rule" his wife. The *command* is: "LOVE your wife, AS CHRIST LOVED the Church. . . ."

It is a common misconception that love is only an emotion or a "feeling." Rather, love is a lasting commitment to the welfare of another, evidenced in acts of kindness and concern and carried out even to the extent of losing one's life in their behalf.

Christ reveals this essence of love as action when He says, *"Do unto others as you would have them do to you"* (Matt. 7:12). By this He does not mean striking a bargain: "I'll be fair to you if you'll be fair to me." Yet how many marriages are structured on this false proposition of give and take?

Christ's meaning goes far deeper. Regardless of the actions of others, we are to give of ourselves to them fully, in the way we would *want* them to give of themselves fully for us. He expands this further when he says, "Love your neighbor *as yourself*." Thus He irrevocably links our loving others with *our capacity to love ourselves*. This "love" is not a self-centered interest but a deep appreciation of our own worth as a human being with a capacity for creative living. A husband who "loves himself" in this way will not be threatened by any abilities his wife may have.

The Danish philosopher Kierkegaard reminds us that our neighbor is not just some person in the abstract but the one who is right *next to us*. Thus one's husband, wife, parent, child, is first of all one's neighbor, who is to be loved "as ourselves." He who does not love any one of the family members with whom he lives, no matter how difficult that person may be, *does not really "love" anyone*, no matter how many others he may seem to love. The husband who does not love his wife doesn't love anyone, for he doesn't even love himself. "He who loves his wife, loves himself."

The Old Testament gives us a beautiful picture of God as the Husband of Israel, long-suffering, generous, loving, forgiving (Isa. 54; Eze. 16:1–14; Hos. 2:14–16). Only when the nation rebelled and deserted Him did they bring trouble upon themselves, and He wooed them back and healed them again and again.

In the New Testament Christ is called the Bridegroom of believers, who loved them enough to die in their behalf. Few husbands are called upon to die for their wives, but Christ also provides the example of how to *live* for them. He says: "The kings of the Gentiles exercise lordship over them; and those in authority are called benefactors. But *not so with you*; rather let the greatest among you become as the youngest, and the leader as one who serves. For which is greater, one who sits at table, or one who serves? Is it not the one who sits at table? But *I am among you as one who serves"* (Luke 22:25,26 rsv).

Jesus not only taught this, but practiced it all through His ministry, even stooping down to wash the disciples' feet, saying to them as He did so, "You also ought to wash one another's feet. For I have given you an example. . . ." (John 13:2–16).

The husband who seeks to lead his household well must even be willing to "wash the feet" of his wife and children, humbling himself to perform menial tasks for those he loves. He must not fail to love and serve not only the ideal wife, but the unlovely, unsubmissive, unthankful, complaining wife, for did not Jesus humble Himself to wash the feet of Peter, who denied Him, and even of Judas, who betrayed Him?

A recent example of a husband humbling himself to serve his wife is Conrad Chisholm, whose wife Shirley was aspiring to be a presidential candidate in the United States. Mr. Chisholm took a temporary leave of absence from his regular job to chauffeur his wife around, help research her speeches, and "see that she's fed, clothed, eats on time and gets to her appointments." He said further, "Shirley's the one out there making it, not me. If you are a man—and a mature man—you do everything to maintain your wife's stardom."[9]

Does such a husband lose respect in the eyes of his wife and children? Not at all. Rather, he stands "ten feet tall" in their eyes. For it is a fact that the husband and father who tries to dominate invites rebellion, insubordination and deception from his wife and children, and he often gets it. He makes a mockery of his "leadership." The humility of true greatness, on the other hand, wins their respect, devotion and obedience.

There is another serious aspect to the leadership of the husband and father, which is that he is responsible for the spiritual welfare of each family member. The Bible warns that the man who prevents his wife or daughter from performing her duties to God "will bear *her* iniquity" (Num. 30). And in regard to little children, Jesus says that "whoever causes one of these little ones who believe in me to sin, it would be better for him to have a great millstone fastened round his neck and to be drowned in the depth of the sea.

See that you do not despise one of these little ones; for I tell you that in heaven their angels always behold the face of my Father who is in heaven" (Matt. 18:6,10).

Thus a husband's and father's primary reponsibility is not to make a name for himself and to earn a living but to live close to God in obedience to Him, giving his family an example to follow.

His secondary responsibility is to provide for their physical needs, food, shelter and clothing. This kindly protection and provision is especially needed during the months of his wife's pregnancy and during the breast-feeding years. He should not only provide for her, but stay close to her, keep involved in her interests, help with the baby and give a lift with the chores. Washing dishes and diapering babies does not make a man "effeminate," for even God is shown as an example of a baby-sitter (Num. 11:12; Isa. 66:13).

Such loving attention on the part of the husband will set the pattern in the home. He will be the leader to whom the others look with respect. Participating in his child's life from the moment of birth will help prevent any "communication gap" from developing later. And in helping his wife to continue blossoming as a person while the children are still small, he will benefit most of all. She will not only become a better, more creative mother but will be able to develop into the kind of stimulating person he will enjoy living with after the children are grown and gone.

SUBMISSIVE WIVES

> Wives, submit yourselves to your own husbands, as to the Lord. (Eph. 5:22.)

> Wives, be in subjection to your own husbands, . . . even as Sarah obeyed Abraham, calling him lord. (I Pet. 3:1–6.)

How many wives have choked on those words? Yet it is a clear teaching of the Bible that no amount of "cultural adaptation" can explain away. But is not a wife's first responsibility to God? Yes. And God's first command to the wife is "submit to your husband." There's no getting around it![10]

Submission does not mean being passive, weak. Submission is a positive attitude, an active, willing, voluntary yielding to the desires

of another. The opposite attitude to submission is not strength—
but insubordination, rebellion and resentment. Submission means
desiring to please the man you love, doing things his way rather
than your own way for the joy of pleasing him.

A wife is given to a man to be his helpmeet (Gen. 2:18–24),
and not the other way around. She is to place his career, his needs,
his wishes first. It is her responsibility to encourage his leadership
ability, to affirm his manliness in her children's eyes, to avoid bur-
dening him with family demands for material things so that he
becomes a slave to his job and shortens his life by overwork. She
co-operates with him in permitting him to pursue the career he
wants, even if it means less pay and material sacrifice for the family.
She develops her own creative potentials not for her own selfish
fulfillment but in order to be a better person, and thus a better
wife and mother.

Such a wife is like the ideal wife of Proverbs 31, who had her
priorities right. Although she was a creative, resourceful person
who fully developed her own talents, she kept the interests of her
husband and children first. In doing this, she found *herself* fulfilled.
She encouraged her husband's endeavors and was proud of his
role as a community leader. His trust in her was not misplaced,
and her children were proud of her.

The ideal wife and mother is also a woman who doesn't talk
too much, knowing that "actions speak louder than words." When
she does speak, she has something to say worth listening to: "She
opens her mouth with wisdom, and *in her tongue is the law of
kindness.*" (Prov. 31:26.)

Such a woman becomes qualified for larger service. Deborah,
leader of the Israelites in the time of the judges (Jud. 4 and 5),
earned the title "a mother in Israel," gaining the right to lead a
nation. And her husband, Lapidoth, apparently did not object.

As women we tend to be defensive about the Biblical commands
to be submissive and to be silent at times (I Cor. 14:34,35), because we forget that what we *are* is already speaking loudly. Our
children are learning from us from the moment of birth through far
more than just the words we speak. Our influence in our husbands'

lives is far greater than just through the words we toss out—which they often do not seem to "hear." (Maybe they are not worth hearing?)

The greatest compliment I ever received came one evening from one of my sons when he was nine years old. I had gone to bed early, not feeling well. After a few moments he came into the room and lay down on the bed beside me. "I just love to come into your room," he said, "because there's such peace in here!"

We know our children need food, clothing, that they must brush their teeth, take baths, get to school on time, practice, do their homework. But do we ever realize that they need *peace?* It had never crossed my mind before. Perhaps there are husbands, too, who long for peace in their households, for less hustle and hurry, for fewer words.

Peter says, "Let your adorning be . . . the hidden person of the heart, even the ornament of a gentle and quiet spirit, which is in the sight of God of great price. For after this manner in the old time the holy women also, who *trusted in God* adorned themselves, being in subjection to their own husbands" (I Peter 3:4, 5).

And then Peter adds, "so that if they [the husbands] don't obey God, your manner of life will win them over . . .". The key to winning over even the wicked, domineering husband is not nagging, bickering, fighting, but a quiet yielding, committing the problem to God and giving Him a chance to solve it in the right way. Remember that "a gentle answer turns away wrath" (Prov. 15:1).

Submission is an important Biblical principle for every person to learn to follow, for it contains the secret of true victory. Jesus said, "If anyone takes away your coat, let him have your overcoat too. And whoever compels you to go a mile, go with him two." (Matt. 5:40, 41.) Christ Jesus Himself is the supreme example of submission, even allowing Himself to be killed because it was God's will:

> The ruler of this world is coming. He has no power over me; but *I do as the Father commanded,* so that the world may know that I love the Father. (John 14:30.)

Christ's obedience was not out of weakness before Satan, to whom he submitted at the cross, and it led not to the end of hope but to His resurrection and the hope of salvation for all mankind.

One wife once complained, "I want to submit to my husband, but he won't take the lead. For example, he always brings the bills to me and wants me to take care of all the financial records. I don't want to do it. *He* ought to do it. *He* ought to be the man of the house!"

This woman was being an unsubmissive wife, resenting her husband for his asking her to do something he knew she could do well, and casting judgments on his manhood because he asked it of her. When she realized that the problem was in wanting him to lead *her* way, according to *her* notions, she changed her attitude and submitted to his desires in the matter.

This is really the key to happy relationships between husband and wife. The more the husband loves his wife, the more willingly does she yield to his every wish. The more the wife seeks to please him, the more he loves her. They may not agree in every matter, but she is willing for him to have the final say in any decision. When she respects his judgment, he is more likely to give her ideas thoughtful consideration. Through the years their tastes will become more and more in harmony until, as Longfellow says, "They were so one, none knew who ruled and who obeyed."

OBEDIENT CHILDREN

An infant needs the love and warmth that come from suckling at the mother's breast and her continual nearness for at least the first several months of life.[11] The daddy's love embraces both the breast-feeding baby and his mother, and the baby enjoys the contentment that comes from being carried in Father's strong arms from the first days of life.

When baby's first steps are taken, symbolic of the move away from close attachment to the mother, reassurance is given by daddy's big hand enfolding the little hand, guiding the steps, until the weary toddler finds security on Daddy's shoulder. The father of small children becomes like God, the Good Shepherd, who "gathers the lambs in his arms, carries them in his bosom, and gently leads those who are with young" (Isa. 40:11).

As children grow, they need freedom to follow their individual interests. Small boys often enjoy dolls until others make fun of them. And why should they not play with dolls? It will make them better fathers. To remove dolls from boys is to intimate that fathers should not be involved with their own babies.

Some girls would rather climb trees than play dolls. Teen-age sons make fine cooks if allowed the opportunity, and it is a big help for girls to know something about auto mechanics. There is no danger that these external activities will interfere with their wholesome development in their own sexual roles, in a home where mothers experience childbirth as a pleasant, natural event, babies are breast-fed, and fathers are supportive of the mother and the children.

Unhappy, troublesome children are often those whose parents are in conflict. For if the parents do not really love each other, how can the child be sure that they love him or her? And his or her sexual identity becomes threatened because he identifies too strongly with one parent and develops hostility toward the other sex. Sexual roles become confused in his mind, for he has no adequate pattern to follow.

Because quarreling parents are disobeying God's rules for a home, a child's obedience suffers, for he tends to pit one parent against the other. Such children become unhappy and destructive because they are not adequately restrained and really do not know what their limits are.

A child should never be allowed to speak disrespectfully of either parent, even in a marriage that has been broken, no matter what the parent may have done. Each parent must insist that the children show respect for the other parent. Women especially tend to be at fault in this regard, causing the father to lose respect in the eyes of his children by belittling him behind his back or finding fault with him in public. But for a child to pass judgment on a parent as a person and be disrespectful is deeply harmful *to the child*. He will become a "difficult" child and may lose respect for all legitimate authority.

Children not only need affirmation in loving attention, cuddling when they are little, and an occasional hug and kiss when they are older. They also need discipline. A happy home is one where each person is loved and affirmed, where there are few rules and few infringements on freedom, but where *no* means *no* to the child. Safeguards must be set for children's behavior, and these few "rules" need to provide them with the security of being consistent, for they will test these barriers to the limit. It gives them a great sense of security when they find that these barriers do not yield either to wiles or tantrums for two-year-olds or teens.

All true authority is derived from another and not grasped for oneself. Even Christ said, "I do nothing on my own authority" (John 5:30). His authority over the church was given Him by the Father. In a home, the leadership has been given by God to the husband and father, who is to yield to the authority of Christ. The wife honors her husband's leadership in the home, and the children are under the authority of both parents, learning both from their precept and example.

There have been times when a child's whole world centered around the home. The father's work took place at or near the home, all activity, leisure, worship, education, centered around the "communal" family, and there were many playmates—brothers and sisters and cousins.

Today there are far more opportunities for individual growth and achievement but also greater stress on family relationships. The husband is away long hours, the children are away at school, the wife is active either in her own job or with volunteer activities, for church, P.T.A. or elsewhere when the children are no longer small. When family members lead such divergent lives, friction can more easily develop unless we follow the safe guide for happy homes, with loving husbands, submissive, gentle wives and obedient children. While this is the ideal, and life is seldom ideal, is there any happier way?

The New Family 315

Notes

1. *Time,* "Male and Female: Differences Between Them," March 20, 1972, p. 43.
2. *The Ante-Nicene Fathers* (Grand Rapids: Eerdmans, 1951), Vol. I, p. 20.
3. *Ibid.,* Vol. II, pp. 419 f.
4. *Time, op. cit.*
5. *Biological Rhythms in Psychiatry and Medicine,* Public Health Service Publication No. 2088, 1970.
6. Jean R. Miller and Margaret E. Armstrong, "The Three R's of Marriage: Relationships, Roles, Responsibilities," *The Standard,* February 15, 1973.
7. Ruth Hoppin, *Priscilla: Author of the Epistle to the Hebrews and Other Essays* (Jericho, N.Y.: Exposition Press, 1972).
8. Albert Rosenfeld, "Why Men Die Younger," *Kansas City Star Sunday Magazine,* October 15, 1972.
9. Quoted in *Time,* March 13, 1972, p. 43.
10. Mary MacAdam, *I Found Freedom* (Parlier, Calif.: Bookmates, 1974).
11. Margaret Ribble, *The Rights of Infants,* rev. ed. (New York: Columbia University Press, 1965).

Appendix

Appendix A

SOURCES OF INFORMATION

American Institute of Family Relations, 5287 Sunset Boulevard, Los Angeles, California 90277.

The AIFR is a responsible resource center for all aspects of marriage and family life. A wide range of publications are available on request.

Home Born Baby is a documentary experience of a family-centered natural childbirth, attended by a doctor and nurse-midwife, narrated by the midwife and the parents. It is a beautiful film, with the perineal view showing the gentle delviery of baby and placenta. Available from Vision Quest, 389 Ethel Ave., Mill Valley, Ca. 94941.

International Childbirth Education Association, P.O. Box 5852, Milwaukee, Wisconsin 53220.

The ICEA is a valuable resource agency for all those who want information concerning childbirth education and current trends in childbirth literature and practice.

ICEA Supplies Center, 208 Ditty Building, Bellevue, Washington 98004.

A wide range of books, pamphlets, films and teaching aids on childbirth education, for both lay and professional people, is available from the ICEA Supplies Center.

La Leche League, International, 9616 Minneapolis Avenue, Franklin Park, Illinois 60131.

Women who want counsel in breast-feeding will find valuable help through the literature and staff of the LLL.

BIBLIOGRAPHY

Bradley, Robert A. *Husband-Coached Childbirth.* New York: Harper & Row, 1965.

Cannon, Walter Bradford. *Bodily Changes in Pain, Hunger, Fear and Rage.* 2nd ed. New York: Harper & Row, 1963.

Chong, Dr. and Mrs. Kwong Tek, and Chua, Mr. and Mrs. Wee Hian. *Lovers for Life.* Singapore: The Way Press, 1971.

Deutsch, Ronald M. *The Key to Feminine Response in Marriage.* New York: Ballantine Books, 1968.

Dick-Read, Grantly. *Childbirth Without Fear.* 4th ed. New York: Harper & Row, 1972.

Flanagan, Geraldine Lux. *The First Nine Months of Life.* New York: Simon and Schuster, 1962.

Fromm, Erich. *The Art of Loving.* New York: Harper & Row, 1956.

Haught, Rosemary. *The Holiness of Sex.* 2nd ed. revised. St. Meinrad, Ind.: Abbey Press, 1968.

Hazell, Lester. *Commonsense Childbirth.* New York: Putnam, 1969.

Jacobson, Edmund. *You Must Relax.* New York: McGraw-Hill, 1962.

Josephson, Elmer A. *God's Key to Health and Happiness.* 2nd ed. revised. Wichita: Bible Light Publications, 1972.

Kitzinger, Sheila. *The Experience of Childbirth.* 2nd ed. revised. Middlesex, England: Penguin Books, 1967.

La Leche League. *Mother's in the Kitchen.* Franklin Park, Ill.: La Leche League, 1972.

La Leche League. *The Womanly Art of Breastfeeding.* 2nd ed. revised. Franklin Park, Ill.: La Leche League, 1953.

MacAdam, Mary. *I Found Freedom.* Parlier, Calif: Bookmates, 1974.

Miller, John S. *Childbirth.* New York: Atheneum, 1963.

Montagu, Ashley. *Human Heredity.* Cleveland: World, 1963.

———. *Life Before Birth.* New York: New American Library, 1964.

———. *Prenatal Influences.* Springfield, Ill.: Thomas, 1962.

———. *Touching, The Human Significance of the Skin.* New York: Columbia University Press, 1971.

Newton, Niles. *The Family Book of Child Care.* New York: Harper & Row, 1957.

Pryor, Karen. *Nursing Your Baby.* New York: Harper & Row, 1963.

Ribble, Margaret. *The Rights of Infants.* 2nd ed. revised. New York: Columbia University Press, 1965.

Tanzer, Deborah. *Why Natural Childbirth?* Garden City, N.Y.: Doubleday, 1972.

Trobisch, Walter. *I Loved a Girl.* New York: Harper & Row, 1963.

———. *I Married You.* New York: Harper & Row, 1971.

———. *Please Help Me, Please Love Me, A Christian View of Contraceptives.* Downers Grove, Ill.: Inter Varsity Press, 1970.

Wiedenbach, Ernestine. *Family Centered Maternity Nursing.* 2nd ed. revised. New York: Putnam, 1967.

Appendix B

INSTRUCTIONS FOR MAKING BACK REST

For delivery tables that are not yet equipped with back rests, or for use in a home delivery, the back rest shown in the illustrations can easily be made. The materials needed for this are as follows:

Two pieces of ⅝" (or ¾" or even ½") plywood panel (preferably pine), 24" by 32".
Two pieces of 1" by 2" by 10' pine boards.
Three pairs 3" butt hinges (preferably brass plated) with ⅝" screws.
Four $5/16$" square head bolts 2½" or 3" long.
Two $5/16$" washers for each bolt.
Four wing nuts for $5/16$" bolts.
Small bottle of wood glue.
A handful of 6 penny finish nails.

Equipment needed: saw, hammer, screwdriver, $5/16$" augur bit and brace, and a keyhole saw.

To assemble the back rest:

Diagram A. The top and bottom boards of plywood panel are the same size. One pair of butt hinges will connect the top and bottom boards at the extreme end of the boards later (see instructions below). One pair of each of the other two pairs of butt hinges is to be screwed to each board as shown on Diagram A, 7" from the end and recessed 3" from each side, later (see Diagram G).

Diagram B. Notice that the butt hinges that unite the top and bottom sections extend slightly past the end of these sections as shown at the left in Diagram B. Notice also that the bottom half of the hinges is mounted on the narrow boards that have been secured to the bottom board according to instructions in Diagram C.

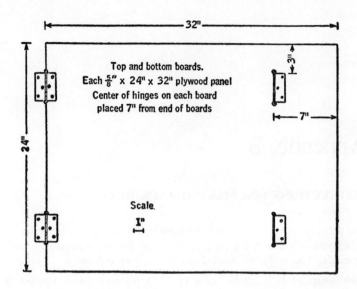

A. Top and bottom boards.

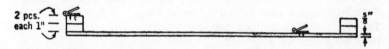

B. Side view of bottom board.

Diagram C. The two pieces of 1″ by 2″ by 10′ pine boards (not ply-wood) are to be cut into lengths shown in Diagram C:

1 piece 1″ x 2″ x 19½″   1 piece 1″ x 2″ x 18″
4 pieces 1″ x 2″ x 17″   4 pieces 1″ x 2″ x 24″

The 24″ pieces are to be screwed (or nailed) to the bottom board of the back rest, two at each end, as shown in Diagram B.

The remaining six pieces are to be assembled as shown on Diagram C, but not until the four 17″ boards have been slotted as shown in Diagram D. (See instructions)

After these four 17″ boards have been slotted, two of them are to be fastened to the 19½″ board, and the other two to the 18″ board, as shown in Diagram C. Any wood glue, and 6 penny box nails can be used. After the outside form (with the 19½″ board) is secured, the other three pieces should be tested inside the frame to be sure they will fit without being too snug. A $\frac{1}{32}''$ play is sufficient for good operation.

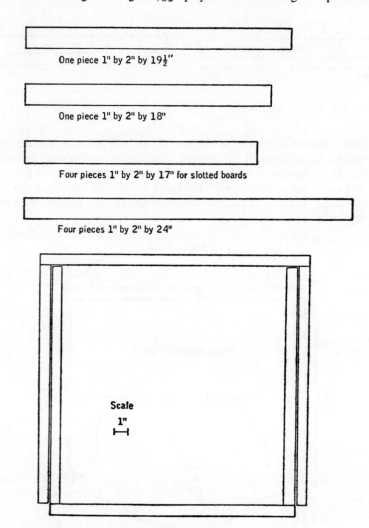

One piece 1" by 2" by $19\frac{1}{2}''$

One piece 1" by 2" by 18"

Four pieces 1" by 2" by 17" for slotted boards

Four pieces 1" by 2" by 24"

Scale
1"
⊢—⊣

C. Detail of 1" by 2" pine boards needed.

Diagram D. The four 1" by 2" by 17" boards are to be slotted as shown on Diagram D. The $\frac{5}{16}''$ slot on each board can be made as follows: Draw a line lengthwise down the center of each board. With a brace and bit drill a $\frac{5}{16}''$ hole at each end of the board with the point of the augur bit placed $2\frac{5}{8}''$ from the end of the board.

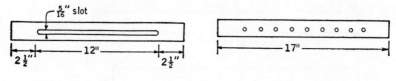

D. Slotted boards.   E. Alternate boards.

Drill a second hole close to the first at one end to make it easier to insert a keyhole saw in the opening. The keyhole saw is used to start the cut lengthwise. A coping saw can be used to start the cut if a key-hole saw is not available. After the initial cut is sufficiently lengthened, any larger saw can be used to complete the 12″ cut on each side of the slot.

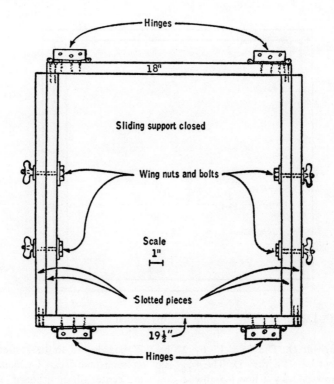

F. Sliding support closed.

Diagram E. If saws are not readily available, a series of $\frac{5}{16}''$ holes spaced $1\frac{1}{2}''$ apart center to center will substitute quite well for the slotted board.

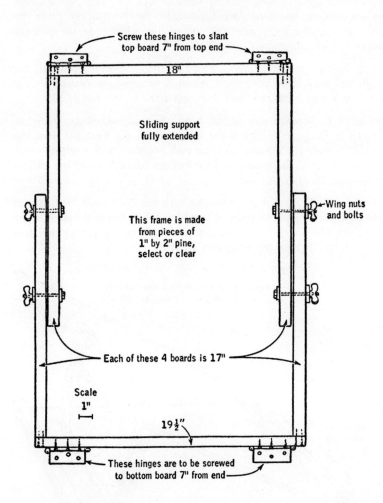

G. Sliding support fully extended.

The only disadvantage is that it takes slightly longer to adjust when in use. However, if the back rest is to be used only occasionally, it would be a very satisfactory method, involving less detail in construction.

Diagram F. Insert the four $\frac{5}{16}''$ square head bolts into the slotted boards as shown in Diagram F., with the washers in place. Fasten them with the $\frac{5}{16}''$ thumb screw pieces (wing nuts). Sufficient pressure can be applied to these wing nuts by hand to lock the back rest securely in the desired position. Any adjustment can be quickly made by loosening all the wing nuts and sliding the supports to the position wanted. (See Diagrams F and G.)

If the boards with holes are used (rather than the slotted boards), the bolts will need to be completely removed to make the desired change of slant in the back rest, and then reinserted in the proper place.

Diagram G. Screw a pair of butt hinges to each end of the frame, as shown in Diagram G. Screw the hinges at the top onto the slant top board 7″ from the top end, as shown on Diagram A. Screw the hinges at the bottom of the frame onto the bottom board 7″ from the end, as shown on Diagram A.

Diagram H. This diagram shows the back rest fully assembled. Notice the position of the three pairs of butt hinges. To change the slant of the back rest, loosen the wing nuts, adjust the upper board to the slant desired, and tighten the wing nuts securely.

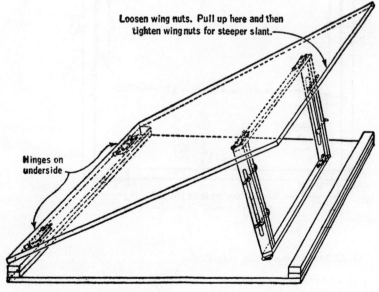

Loosen wing nuts. Pull up here and then tighten wing nuts for steeper slant.

Hinges on underside

H. The back rest assembled.

Diagrams I and J. To close the back rest, remove the bolts and wing nuts. The supports will then fold to the inside. A hook and eye will be convenient for securing the back rest in the closed position, as indicated on these two diagrams.

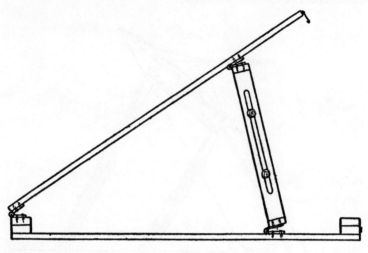

I. Side view, open.

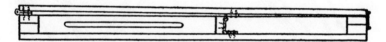

J. Side view, closed. Supports folded inside.

Diagram K. The back rest may be finished with paint or varnish, to make it scrubbable. It can be fastened to the delivery table with a heavy canvas strap, like that of a strong traveling case or the safety strap in a car. This is passed under the table and buckled securely in place. Or, if it is not possible to pass the strap under the table, it can be snapped around any firm projection on each side of the delivery table, to hold the back rest in place.

A 2″ or 3″ thick foam-rubber pad 24″ x 32″, covered with rubber or plastic sheeting and a removable fitted cotton pillowcase, makes a good backing. This can be snapped onto the top of the board to prevent shifting. (See Diagram K.)

Another method is to make a contour sheet with overlap of six inches. The top section can be slipped over the top of the back rest to hold the pad in place. For additional comfort, a pillow can be placed under the mother's head and shoulders. A supply of fresh pillowcases or contour sheets should be constantly available.

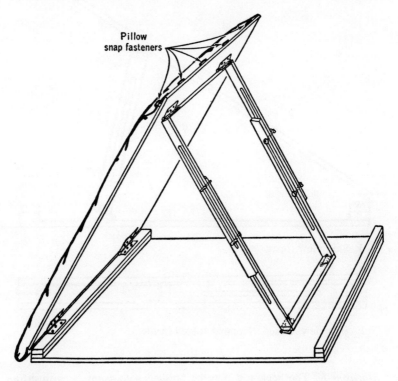

Pillow
snap fasteners

K. Back rest with pad.

When the back rest is in use, the stirrups of the delivery table should be kept low but with the mother's knees supported slightly above the level of her hips, so that she will not have a tendency to "slide down" off the back rest.

Index

Abdomen, lower, tightening and pressure in, as sign of labor, 126
Abortion, 30, 169, 170, 171, 172, 173
Abstinence, as form of birth control, 27
Adrenalin, release of oxytocin inhibited by, 289
Africa, couvade practiced in, 165
Afterbirth, 56, 127; delivery of, 266–267
Agrippina, 170
Ainus of Japan, 165
American Institute of Family Relations, 276
American Public Health Association, 217
Analgesia, 163, 195, 204, 217, 218, 258
Anesthesia, 58, 82, 116, 163, 195, 204, 213, 217–222 *passim*, 258, 272; spinal, 220, 221
Anoxia, 216, 217
Anthropology, 59, 66; evidences from, for easier childbirth, 163–177
Apgar, Virginia, 217
Apōthlibō, defined and translated, 184
Aquila, 193
Arab women, and childbirth, 66
Armstrong, Margaret E., quoted, 302
Asphyxia, postnatal, 212, 213, 216
Atelectasis, 212, 213
August, Ralph W., 227, 228; quoted, 228
Augustus Caesar, 170
Authorized Version, 186, 193

Autosuggestion, 130, 226
Aztec women, role of, 165

Baby, *see* Infant
Back rest, 244–245; instructions for making, 321–328
Bakwin, Harry, quoted, 245
Basanidzō, defined and translated, 186
Basques of Spain, 165
Bible, teaching of, on childbirth, 61, 63–71 *passim*, 97–105 *passim*, 116, 117, 178–198 *passim*; *see also* New Testament; Old Testament
"Biblical Teaching Concerning Labor and Childbirth" (Wessel), xix
Birth, *see* Childbirth
Birth canal, 43, 53, 54, 55, 127, 142, 143, 149
Birth climax, 69, 223–224, 270–274
Birth control, methods of, 27–30
"Birthstool," 167, 243
Bisacodyl (suppository) patients, 207
Blake, Florence, 245; quoted, 222, 246, 247
Blood transfusion, 163
Bordeaux, Jean, quoted, 226, 227
Bradley, Robert A., 237, 249; quoted, 236, 238, 250
Brassiere, nursing, 151
Breaking suction, in breast-feeding, 288
"Breast-Eze," 290
Breast-feeding, 267–270, 279–297; benefits of, to mother, 280, 281; and engorgement, 290–292; instructions for, 150–151; and

329

332   Index

73 74 75 76 77 10 9 8 7 6 5 4 3 2 1